WHITELOTUS

Holistic Cosmetic Acupuncture

The Natural Guide to Rejuvenating
Facial Acupuncture

Antony Kingston with Kamila Kingston

Cover design by Anthony Kingston©

Original illustrations/ Photographs by Anthony Kingston©

ISBN: 978-0-646-82802-2

White Lotus Beauty

21/222 Chester Pass Road, Walmsley, WA, 6330
www.whitelotusbeauty.com
www.whitelotus.com.au

Notice to the Reader

Table of Contents

introduction...1

Chapter 1: A Short History Of Cosmetic Acupuncture 3

Chapter 2: How Does Cosmetic Acupuncture Work? 5

How Does it Work From a Traditional Chinese Medicine (Tcm) Perspective
....5
How Does it Work From a Scientific Perspective? 7
Research on Deeper Needling and Alternative Mechanisms of Action 11
Subcision Aka Circling the Dragon...13

Chapter 3: Setting Up Your Cosmetic Acupuncture Clinic 15

The Cosmetic Acupuncture Marketplace 15
Therapeutic Claims in Advertising...18
Ethics..18
Preparing the Clinic Space...19
Packages of Treatment and Treatment Timing...20
Key Cautions and Contra Indications 22
Pretreatment Advice for the Client 23
Post Treatment Procedure...24

Chapter 4: Traditional Chinese Facial Diagnosis 26

Colours of the face...28
Regions of the Face and the Significance of Lines and Blemishes in these
areas 29

Chapter 5: Facial Cosmetic Acupuncture Needling Techniques.................35

Guiding Principles of FCA Needling..35
Types of Needles..36
Needle Retention Times 37
Threading 37
Subcision 39
Lifting and Pinning 39
Intradermal Acupuncture Needles...40
Acupuncture Points and Ashi Points 41
Lip Enhancement 42
Distal Points...44
The Influence of Skin Colour on Needling Depth.......................................44

Chapter 6: Chinese Medicine Pattern Differentiation and Constitutional
Treatment 46

Wrinkles..46

Sagging Skin 48

Scars 49

Acne 52

Vitiligo 55

Chapter 7: Step by Step Instructions for Specific Cosmetic Issues 57

Sagging Neck and Neck Lines.. 57
Marionette Lines (Vertical lines from the chin to the corner of the mouth)
.... 58

Mouth Frown Lines (Vertical lines next to the mouth).................... 58
Nasolabial Folds (The corner of the nose to the corner of the mouth)....... 58
Sagging Cheeks 59
Vertical Lip Lines (Vertical lines above and below the mouth) 59
Horizontal Lines Below the Eye 61
Bags Below the Eyes 61
Crow's Feet 63
Horizontal Lines on the Bridge of the Nose............................ 63
Frown Lines (Vertical Lines Between the Eyebrows)................ 63
Drooping Eyelids... 63
Forehead Lines (Horizontal Lines Across the Forehead) 64

Chapter 8: Complementary Treatments 65

Why Use Complementary Treatments? 65
When to Use Complementary Treatments? 65
Acupressure 66
Jade Rollers... 67
Jade Gua Sha 67
Cosmetic Cupping.. 68
Micro-needle Rollers.. 68
Summary of the Order of Treatment................................... 69

Appendixes 70

Appendix A: Products Used During Treatments...................... 70
Appendix B: Traditional External Application of Chinese Herbs 72
Appendix C: Taking Before and After Photos 73
Appendix D - Other Publications by the Author..................... 74

Introduction

Anthony and Kamila founded White Lotus Cosmetic Acupuncture in Brisbane Australia in 2007. At the time it was the only specialist cosmetic acupuncture clinic in Australia and one of only several in the world. The clinic was the result of many years studying and practicing in Australia, China, Malaysia and Singapore. This book is the result of their combined 30 years practicing and teaching the ancient beauty rituals of the Far East to audiences all around the world.

This passion and teaching has spurned a global business which provides education and equipment to share the ancient cosmetic secrets of China in clinics and homes across the world.

The book is very specifically designed for acupuncturists with a passion for cosmetic practice. Many books on acupuncture facial rejuvenation pad the content with basic theories of Chinese Medicine. This book includes the traditional theory which Kamila and Anthony are well versed in but only where it pertains directly to the practice and results you can achieve with Facial Cosmetic Acupuncture (FCA). In other words it has to be relevant. This knowledge of TCM is combined with a unique perspective derived from years working with mainstream beauty therapists and aestheticians.

FCA should never be separated from the ancient theories which guide every needle insertion. Neither should it ignore the explanations of modern science which prove what the ancient Chinese already knew.

Through diagrams, photographs and detailed explanations this book attempts to take the reader on a journey to discover how FCA really works and how we can best serve our clients in its application.

Throughout this book the use of acupuncture for cosmetic enhancement on the face is referred to as Facial Cosmetic Acupuncture (FCA). In many places this is not the preferred terminology and terms like 'Acupuncture Facial Rejuvenation','Facial Enhancement Acupuncture', 'Constitutional Facial Acupuncture' and simply 'Facial acupuncture' are more common. There are various reasons for this. In some areas the local licensing bodies prescribe preferred terms for use. In other areas a particular term was popularised by a prominent proponents of FCA to differentiate their techniques.

It is best to check with your local body as to which term is best to advertise with in your specific area.

The book is broadly divided into two parts, the theory, and the practice though there is plenty of overlap. This is done deliberately. You will miss a lot if you skip the theory, however in future you may simply want to quickly refer back to check a particular technique. In this way the books becomes not only a great reference book but also a practical day to day work book.

Chapter 1

A Short History of Cosmetic Acupuncture

The history of applying Chinese medicine for cosmetic purposes is long. The second book (treatise five) of the *Huang Di Nei Jing* (Yellow Emperor's Classic of Internal Medicine) mentions the use of Chinese medicine to treat the skin and hair. The Systemised Canon of Acupuncture and Moxibustion, *Zhen Ju Jia Yi Ying* (282 AD) alludes to the use of acupuncture needles to improve the faces appearance. Sun Si Miao's (581-682 AD) classical text, *Bei Ji Qian Jin Yao Fang* (Essential Prescriptions Worth a Thousand Liang in Gold for Every Emer-gency) lists 105 formulas with cosmetic applications.

This history above is not to be confused with direct references to needle insertion solely for cosmetic purposes. It is surprising how often you see articles and web-sites that state FCA was first recorded in ancient texts thousands of years ago. This is indirectly true but the process had little in common with how FCA is now practiced. Cosmetic benefits were usually the indirect results of treatments to im-prove general health.

FCA as we now know it now is a relatively recent phenomenon though it draws from and is inseparable from the ancient theories of Chinese Medicine. Verbal reports from doctors in China expressed to the author relate that in 1974 Mao Zedong instigated a group to investigate the effectiveness of applying acupuncture for cosmetic purposes. This group's work was said to have continued until 1980 when the project was discontinued. Unfortunately these reports have prov-en hard to corroborate with reliable written evidence.

Whether this group existed or not it is true that during this time a great deal of research was done into the use of acupuncture for facial rejuvenation, weight loss, cellulite, stretch marks and breast enhancement amongst others. Western students returning from China increasingly returned with new cosmetic tech-niques they applied in their clinics. Simultaneously Doctors emigrated from Chi-na to the USA, UK, Australia and Canada brought with them a variety of cosmetic acupuncture practices.

By the 1990,s FCA was well established in some parts of China. This was highlighted by a 1996 Chinese study of 300 cases of FCA. The research overwhelm-ingly supported the efficacy of the techniques. [1]

There has been much research into acupuncture for cosmetic purposes since. So much in fact that a whole chapter is dedicated to it. Reading this chapter is not required in order to effectively practice the techniques taught here but it will enhance your understanding of FCA. Additionally it will allow you to better ex-plain to your clients how FCA works in a language they can understand.

Chapter 2

How Does Cosmetic Acupuncture Work?

HOW DOES IT WORK FROM A TRADITIONAL CHINESE MEDICINE (TCM) PERSPECTIVE

The most important point that differentiates the TCM perspective from the scientific understanding is that the TCM pattern involves the whole person and the whole body. The scientific explanation is localised to the structures of the skin.

The fact that the TCM understanding of FCA includes the whole body is a key reason FCA can and should never be divorced from TCM theory. Being able to benefit the whole person as part of a localised cosmetic treatment increases the benefits and leads to longer lasting results. It is also a key differentiating factor between FCA and other cosmetic treatments available on the market.

The first and most obvious way FCA achieves results is by improving qi and blood circulation. The seems very obvious and is not so different from the common claim of increasing microcirculation in western cosmetic practices. This will occur naturally with all types of FCA and needs little further discussion.

FCA also raises qi (energy) to reduce sagging. This is again true and is more noticeable with some techniques than others. It is also more relevant where the predominant issue concerning the client is sagging. This sagging is usually of the skin on the cheeks, jowls, neck and under the eyes. It can also be pertinent to sagging of the eyelids especially the upper eyelids which are now sometimes treated surgically in western medicine.

FCA balances yin and yang. All acupuncture performs this function so this is more of an advertising slogan than a useful diagnostic or treatment principle. Some teachers go so far as to equate yin and yang with collagen and elastin respectively. This sounds fascinating printed on a flyer (which is in itself useful) but has little real relevance to how the treatments work.

The points above describe how FCA improves facial appearance from a very simplified TCM perspective.

It becomes much more interesting when you combine the question of how the treatments work with detailed TCM facial diagnosis. Using these facial diagnosis techniques each wrinkle, blemish or area of sagging on the face represents the health of an underlying TCM organ. To put it another way each wrinkle on the face is directly caused by an imbalance in one of the key organs (abetted by age of course and its effects on organ health).

If a wrinkle is caused by a disharmony of an internal organ then directly assisting this organ with distal points, Chinese herbs and other TCM practices should start to reduce the appearance of the wrinkle.

The next step is the part a lot of practitioners do not immediately grasp. If a wrinkle is caused by an imbalance in the underlying organ controlling that part of the face then by reducing the appearance of the wrinkle you can also improve the health of the underlying organ.

This is in a nutshell how FCA produces results from a TCM perspective. You target the wrinkles which are the manifestations of the organ disharmony directly with FCA. You also target the cause of the wrinkles with distal points and herbs to rebalance the body. In this way you can treat both root and branch in a very focused way. Each wrinkle or blemish has a very specific diagnosis and pattern you are improving.

This relationship between wrinkles and the internal organs is not only about the treatments themselves. It is also about improving your diagnosis to create better treatments.

I have always used four simple lines to drill this into my students.

- By diagnosing the face you diagnose the body
- By diagnosing the body you diagnose the face
- By treating the face you treat the body
- By treating the body you treat the face

A real life example can help illustrate this. One of the most common wrinkles you will be asked to treat is the 'suspended sword'. This is the deep single vertical line that many people develop between the eyebrows.

In TCM facial diagnosis this area of the the face and particularly this line is related to the liver and most often to liver qi stagnation. When you see this line on your clients face you can immediately start thinking about liver qi stagnation as a potential pattern. You can then use other diagnostic skills such as pulse, tongue and questioning to confirm this diagnosis and look for other patterns.

Assuming your diagnosis is confirmed you can then treat the liver qi stagnation directly with acupuncture points on the liver channel and Chinese herbal formulas such as Xiao Yao San. This will start to make the person feel better and directly target the cause of the wrinkle.

Simultaneously you can target the 'suspended sword' with localised needling techniques such as 'threading' which will be explained later. This will directly target the wrinkle by reducing qi and blood stagnation in the local area and importantly help circulate liver qi in the whole body again assisting the cause of the wrinkle.

It is this two way street of treating the localised wrinkles to benefit the whole person while treating the whole person to benefit the wrinkle that makes FCA so effective.

HOW DOES IT WORK FROM A SCIENTIFIC PERSPECTIVE?

Does FCA increase Microcirculation and lymphatic drainage?

Simple answer yes it does. Virtually any form of massage or stimulation of the skin will at least minimally increase both. Realistically this is more useful for advertising copy than a genuinely unique mechanism for the effectiveness of FCA. We need to dig deeper to see what is really going on.

Does FCA achieve Results through Collagen Induction?

The ambiguous answer is yes and no. FCA produces a small part of its results through collagen induction but if this was the only mechanism then FCA would be a very ineffective cosmetic treatment compared to others.

Collagen is such a buzz word in the cosmetic industry that it is no wonder it is so often used to explain the effectiveness of FCA. At present you can take collagen in almost any form. You can apply it topically, inject it and even drink it assuming you are happy to ignore the fact that your stomach acid breaks it down almost instantly.

At the time of writing, no studies have been done to measure the increase in collagen induction following a treatment with FCA on humans.

One 2015 study on mice found that acupuncture may protect the skin from UV radiation damage, decrease wrinkle formation, reduce loss of epidermal thickness and reduce the degradation of collagen fibres in the skin (note: the wording "reduce degradation" rather than induce new collagen). [2]

This study is too limited to provide much evidence of the affects of FCA on collagen induction in humans but studies on other forms of skin needling can shed some light on this subject.

Micro-needling is a subject I have a lot of experience with having used and taught with these devices for over a decade. There is a lot more research on these devices as the commercial motivation is much stronger. This research gives us a clearer insight into how the collagen induction process works.

Micro-needling is the use of small hand-held rollers that usually contain between 180 and 340 tiny needles (micro-needles). Each needle is between 0.5mm and 1.5 millimetres long. [3] When a micro-needle roller is rolled across the skin 15 times it produces an average of 215 punctures per square centimetre. [4]

To measure collagen induction, skin biopsies are taken and collagen content in the skin before and after the treatment. Following a micro-needling treatment an average increase in collagen of approximately 206% has been recorded. [5]

Some participants in these studies have even demonstrated up to a 1,000% increased collagen induction.[5] It is understood that this collagen is produced as a result of the mild trauma that activates the physiological wound healing cascade. [6]

This clearly demonstrates that some forms of needling are capable of increasing collagen induction in the skin. Unfortunately the number of punctures made by a micro-needling roller makes it very difficult to speculate how much collagen a single acupuncture needle can produce. If the wound-healing cascade is indeed the cause of the collagen induction then this strongly suggests that more punctures will induce more collagen. FCA treatments which employ between ten and thirty facial needles will therefore be far less effective than treatments such as micro needling at inducing collagen.

Additionally when these micro-needling skin biopsies are studied it has been shown that because the needle punctures are so close together a complete new matrix of collagen and elastin are laid down. Individual acupuncture needles with their much greater spacing between insertion points will never be able to accomplish this feat.

Studies using micro-needling rollers with needles up to 1.5 millimetres long have also shown that collagen induction only takes place up to 0.6 millimetres into the skin. The new collagen forms directly on the border between the epidermis and the dermis. [5] Most FCA practitioners typically insert needles much deeper than this. Even shallow needle 'threading' techniques that pass under wrinkles penetrate the skin by at least several millimetres.

The question then becomes whether practitioners who employ deeper needling techniques on the face are missing the point as collagen induction only takes place when needling very shallowly. Longer needles will of course also induce some collagen as they pass through the superficial levels of the skin, but penetration beyond 0.6 millimetres into the skin would seem to be unnecessary if the goal was collagen induction alone.

Ultimately if the goal of FCA was simply collagen induction then your clients would be much better off with a micro-needling treatment or one of the numerous other cosmetic treatments that can measurably induce much larger quantities of collagen. Some of these other cosmetic treatments are of course far more deeply invasive than micro-needling and are best avoided but the fact remains that for FCA to be as effective as practices such as micro-needling something else must be going on.

Fortunately there is as we will see in the next section.

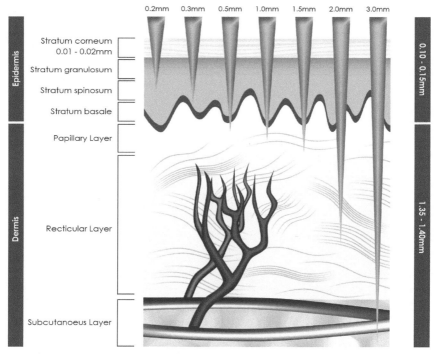

Image 1: This depicts the different layers of the skin that an acupuncture needles passes through.

Some important points to note for our purposes are

1. *The Stratum corneum: This is the surface layer of the epidermis. It is this layer which provides the skins water proof barrier. As you can see it is only between 0.01-0.02mm thick. Very short needles can be used to puncture it and increase transdermal absorption. This is a key reason for only using natural non toxic products on the skin when performing any form of skin needling.*

2. *The Epidermis: The epidermis is only between 0.1 and 0.15mm thick. The needles must pass through this layer into the dermis to stimulate fibroblast activity which initiate collagen induction.*

3. *The Dermis: Lying below the epidermis the dermis comprises the majority of the thickness of the skin. Minor trauma to this area caused by the needles causes the fibroblasts to induce collagen as part of the wound healing cascade. The majority of this collagen induction occurs in the Papilliary layer up to 0.6mm deep, on the border of the epidermis.*

4. *Fibroblasts (not pictured): Fibroblasts are cells located in the dermis which synthesize collagen. They have become something of a 'holy grail' of the cosmetic industry in recent decades. Production of new collagen is a key goal in creating younger looking skin.*

RESEARCH ON DEEPER NEEDLING AND ALTERNATIVE MECHANISMS OF ACTION

Conducting a brief review of the literature will reveal at least 27 studies on FCA over the last 15 years.[7] Several of these studies suggest alternative explanations for FCA's effectiveness.

The most important mechanism that emerges is that FCA influences the muscles in ways not previously studied. Penetration of needles into these muscles may be a key part of the mechanism of action of FCA.

As background it is important to understand the early research on acupuncture for Bells Palsy. This research showed that acupuncture needles can improve muscle tone in the face. A 2015 review included 14 randomised controlled trials on Bells Palsy and concluded that acupuncture can assist both the paralysis and the **muscle weakness** caused by Bells Palsy. [8]

Loss of elasticity in the facial (mimetic) muscles and muscle weakness in the facial muscles is widely considered an inevitable part of ageing and thus contributes to the appearance of ageing in the face. [9] What is often not understood is that facial muscles gradually shorten and straighten with age due to increased resting muscle tone. [8]

A 2007 study effectively showed that FCA can restore mimetic muscle tone. This was measured by an MRI which showed changes in the contour of the facial muscles. [9] In 2013 this idea was further supported by a study which employed multiple sessions of FCA over several weeks to improve mimetic muscles and facial elasticity. [10] Moire topography was used to measure changes after the FCA sessions. A small but noticeable difference was recorded (First used in 1970 Moire topography is a widely used technique to evaluate topographical changes in the the human body. In this study it was employed to evaluate the changes in contour lines in the cheek and perioral region). These studies suggest that FCA may be able to restore muscle tone to a more 'youthful' state and change the actual facial shape.

Several further studies suggest that this relaxing of the muscles of the face may have other benefits. In 2008 a study speculated that drying of the skin on the face may be caused by heat generated by tight facial muscles. [11] This heat becomes greater with age as the resting muscle tone increases. The study went on to show that FCA may be able to reduce this heat and in this way slow or even reduce the signs of ageing caused by dryness of the skin. This idea has been further supported by a 2013 study showing that FCA using acupuncture points on the face increased oil and water content on the face after treatment. [12]

It appears that FCA may reduce the resting facial muscle tone that naturally increases with age. This can then contribute to beneficial changes in facial shape. By increasing relaxation and elasticity of these muscles it may also reduce the heat produced by the muscles, reducing skin dryness which is associated with wrinkle formation.

Importantly if at least part of the mechanism of action lies in penetration of the deeper muscles of the face then acupuncture needling has a distinct advantage over more superficial cosmetic techniques such as micro-needling that focus solely on collagen induction.

SUBCISION AKA CIRCLING THE DRAGON

One further human study will be of special interest to practitioners who use 'threading' techniques to needle directly under wrinkles and scars. In ancient times needling under scars in this way was referred to as 'circling the dragon'.

The study employed a tri beveled syringe. The syringe was inserted under a depressed scar and then manipulated. The analysis of the skin showed that the syringe had increased collagen induction in the area. Additionally and more importantly it had separated the scar tissue from the healthy tissue below literally allowing the depressed scar to 'pop up'. [13]

The study coined the term 'subcision' which is now commonly used in modern FCA research.

The collagen induction was expected as all forms of skin needling will induce some collagen induction due to the trauma created. What was more interesting to the researchers was that the needling seemed to be able to break the bonds connecting the scar tissue to healthy tissue below. This allowed it to effectively raise depressions in the skin such as depressed (hypotrophic) scars and potentially wrinkles.

This mechanism, as much as any other, may explain why threading under wrinkles is so effective. It would also explain why wrinkles appear to rise so noticeably during and after treatment.

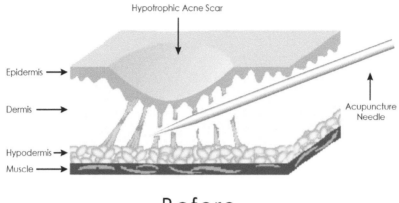

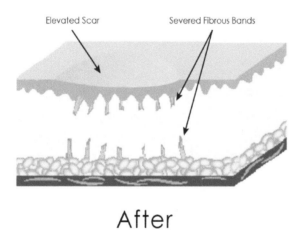

Image 2: Depicts the process by which subcision breaks the bands below scars to allow hypotrophic scars and potentially wrinkles to rise after treatments.

Chapter 3

Setting up Your Cosmetic Acupuncture Clinic

THE COSMETIC ACUPUNCTURE MARKETPLACE

In our courses over the years in addition to Chinese medicine practitioners we have taught Doctors, Nurses and chiropractors all of which are qualified to practice acupuncture. We have also spent a large amount of time training Aestheticians, Beauticians, Cosmetic Nurses and Cosmetic Dentists in micro needling and other traditional Chinese cosmetic practices.

This advice below is specifically aimed at acupuncturists trained from a TCM background. It is based on our experience working in both traditional acupuncture clinics and modern aesthetic clinics.

When you commence offering FCA there are two main streams from which you can or will draw clients. The first is your traditional client base. They have been exposed to acupuncture before. They understand some parts of the diagnosis process and are especially interested in the natural approach to aesthetic improvement. These are the clients you are familiar with and you should be able to manage them easily.

Depending on your marketing and positioning in the market, the second group you may attract are those who spend a lot of time exploring the range of cosmetic treatments available. They may be less familiar with a genuinely natural approach to beauty. Many will have been sold the idea that a dollop of organic aloe vera in a beauty cream represents the zenith of natural cosmetic experiences.

These clients can become excellent converts over time. I notice though that many trained acupuncturists often struggle to understand and convert these clients. I feel this is largely due to a lack of understanding of the aesthetic industry and the competition you are now facing if you wish to compete in this marketplace.

We learnt this the hard way many years ago when we opened our first solely cosmetic clinic. It was rapidly featured in several high profile magazines and then on national television. This attracted a totally different audience to that with which we had been accustomed. Popular magazine 'Well Being' in particular retitled one of my articles "Better than Botox". This bought in a wave of clients with very different expectations and created a steep learning curve.

If you want to effectively attract and retain these clients you must familiarise yourself with the industry and learn the vocabulary your new clients are used to. I have spent quite some time earlier in the book explaining the scientific processes through which FCA works. The text and diagram also focus on the different levels of the skin and how collagen is actually inducted.

This is not only there as an explanation for your understanding. It is there to provide exposure to the vocabulary your clients will expect you to possess. This is not instead of your traditional Chinese diagnosis, it is in addition to that knowledge.

The aesthetic industry is a much faster moving industry than the acupuncture industry. Beauty salons have to stay constantly alert to the latest developments in aesthetics. Clients are always approaching them looking for the next 'silver bullet' in the fight against the inevitable signs of ageing.

The beauty industry is also a hugely popular career choice. It has low barriers to entry and is a passion for a large percentage of the population.

Combine these two factors with the huge amount of money involved and it is not surprising that the beauty industry is one of the most competitive and trend dominated marketplaces in the world.

I often say to my students "FCA is such a wonderful and effective therapy but if you can't market it no one will benefit from your skills". In the past I used to receive some resistance to this comment as though selling your skills was in some way impure and lessened the integrity of the art. Thankfully as the years have passed this attitude has subsided and 'how do I market my clinic?' is actually one of the most common questions I am asked at the end of seminars.

If you are genuinely interested in improving the marketing of your clinic then study how the beauty industry markets. Look at the top line day spas and high end clinics. They have usually spent millions on marketers and designers and their presentation is some of the best in the world. Studying their materials allows you to benefit from their marketing expertise. In the beauty industry great presentation and marketing are not a bonus they are simply expected.

Fortunately this message is being heard. I have seen many of my ex students build up brilliant clinics that compete with and often better the best in the beauty industry. I recently noticed an acupuncturists who attended one of my seminars many years ago is now the residential acupuncturist at Harrods in London. His marketing and presentation is sublime and the fees he now commands are intimidating. This is what is expected at the top end of the aesthetic industry.

I touched earlier on the need to learn a new vocabulary. This is vital. Many of your new clients will be very familiar with the processes of collagen induction, transdermal absorption, correct exfoliation etc. It is distinctly embarrassing if you are holding yourself up as a cosmetic expert and your client knows more about the industry than you do. They begin to doubt your expertise.

At very least you should thoroughly review the anatomy of the skin and gain a basic understanding of the other cosmetic therapies you are competing against. Common questions you will receive in clinic will include.

1. How does FCA compare to microblading?
2. How long after microdermal abrasion can I receive FCA?
3. Can I have FCA at the same time as Botox?
4. You say FCA will detoxify my skin does this mean my expensive Botox treatment won't last as long???

Only with a thorough understanding of your new industry can you hope to answer these questions and convince your new clients you are worth listening too.

THERAPEUTIC CLAIMS IN ADVERTISING

Most practitioners who have an online presence or perform regular marketing activities will already be aware that we must be careful not to claim to 'treat' or especially to be able to 'cure' any recognised illness without very strong scientific evidence of the effectiveness. This evidence is almost always lacking for acupuncture treatments.

Unintentionally making these claims can lead to actions against you. Websites of acupuncturists and other alternative practitioners are increasingly being monitored by private groups who feel they are doing a public service to have these offending websites shut down.

What many of you may not be aware of is that many cosmetic conditions are actually considered recognised illnesses. So while you may be able to make multiple claims about the effectiveness of your treatments against wrinkles or sagging skin (within reason) you must be careful if making any claims about assisting scars, acne or hair loss. Claiming to treat or cure any of these can constitute a therapeutic claim. More obviously conditions such as vitiligo and rosacea are also considered medical conditions.

Regulations will vary based on your country of practice but alway seek advice about this if you are unsure of your content.

ETHICS

It is a given that you should follow all ethical practices common to regular acupuncture. These include amongst others maintaining confidentiality, listening attentively and referring where appropriate.

Additionally be very aware that some FCA clients who come to you may have poor self image or even psychological issues resulting from very low self-esteem. In this case no amount of FCA is going to improve their sense of well being. These clients should be referred where necessary to someone more qualified to assist them. This is better for you as a practitioner as well as for them.

Remember to always emphasise the positive in a person's face as well as the problem areas. I have seen some practitioners make their clients thoroughly dependent on them by constantly emphasising all their issues that only they can fix. This is not a healthy relationship.

It is better for a person to leave your consultation feeling good about themselves and looking forward to positive change in the future than to make money on peoples misery about their appearance. This would be a very depressing environment to work in.

PREPARING THE CLINIC SPACE

All practices and protocols required to meet the standards of an acupuncture clinic in your local area should be followed. These are available from your local authority if this is your first clinic.

From a purely FCA point of view there are a few things you need to consider.

Lighting is incredibly important. Generally your clients will be more visually orientated and so will not appreciate dark, gloomy rooms. More importantly it is vital you can see their skin very clearly to better assess it. It is also important as good lighting allows you to accurately judge the borders of scars and the depth of needling.

Natural light is best but failing that a beauticians lamp can be of great assistance. It not only provides additional light but magnifies the skin to help you with the diagnostic process.

If you are applying any solutions or products to your clients skin have them on prominent display. If a client is coming to you for FCA the chances are they are very aware of what goes on their skin and will want full disclosure about the ingredients in everything you use.

This also applies to the acupuncture needles which should always be removed from their sterile packaging in front of the client (without drawing too much attention to the needles for needle phobics). This way the client can be sure they are sterile and single use.

Always have a small preparation area in your clinic with a mirror. Many of your clients will want to check their appearance and do their hair before leaving.

Finally if you plan to take before and after photos which are discussed in the appendix make sure you have an area set up for this with consistent lighting.

PACKAGES OF TREATMENT AND TREATMENT TIMING

In practice FCA can either be performed as an ongoing treatment or in predetermined packages. A discount is usually applied to the packages for upfront payment.

This eases the financial burden on clinics but more importantly it ensures clients commit to the time frame you require to achieve genuine results.

The original protocols we observed in China set out packages of 15 treatments over a 3-4 week period. This required the client to attend the clinic 2-3 times a week.

This is not generally the most effective way to work with Western clients. The problems with this approach are two fold. They are patient compliance and the pace of deeper constitutional change.

For most clients in the modern world, three times a week is simply too large a commitment. The world is very busy. We often have clients who are only flying in for the day. They need to see you on the days when they are in town. For other clients it is too large a financial commitment every week. The packages must be practical for their situation to help them achieve results.

Just as importantly one of the huge advantages of FCA over other cosmetic treatments is the ability to create genuine constitutional change. This takes place through pattern diagnosis, FCA, constitutional acupuncture and where possible herbal medicine. It is very hard to make real long lasting changes to a clients health in only 3-4 weeks.

To give an example. If you have a client with sagging skin and an underlying pattern of Spleen qi deficiency (weak digestion). You will achieve far better results if you can see them weekly for 10-15 weeks. During this time you can apply FCA, distal points and potentially herbal medicine to address the underlying Spleen qi deficiency. Fifteen weeks allows more time for this deep constitutional change to take place than the same number of treatments performed over 3-4 weeks. If you can improve the underlying spleen qi deficiency that contributes to the sagging skin simultaneously then the FCA will produce far more long lasting results.

For a smaller package the minimum number of treatments I recommend is six treatments over six weeks. Any less than this and you will not see the same substantial results in reducing wrinkles and other signs of ageing. Bear in mind that the skin completely regenerates itself approximately every 27 days. Ideally you want to work through at least one full cycle of regeneration and preferably two, so eight sessions over eight weeks is even better.

The previous discussion of packages does not mean that clients will not see results after one session. Quite the contrary. After one session clients should see a general tightening of the skin, reduction in swelling and fluid retention especially around the eyes and an improvement in skin tone.

It is to make longer lasting changes to sagging, wrinkles and other blemishes that requires more time. These changes need to take place at a deeper level.

Follow up treatments can be performed in packages 1-3 months later. In practice many clients simply choose to continue with the treatments long term and continue to attend weekly, fortnightly or monthly as their budget and commitments allow.

KEY CAUTIONS AND CONTRA INDICATIONS

1. Pregnancy: FCA is better reserved for after pregnancy and all efforts focused on the health of the mother and child.

2. Vertigo and dizziness: This depends on the TCM pattern differentiation but in general it is not a good idea to dramatically increase blood flow to the head of a client with vertigo unless you are very sure of your diagnosis.

3. Severe high blood pressure: Again this could exasperate the condition.

4. Severe migraines or headaches: Although a contraindication this depends on your pattern differentiation as many headaches will benefit from FCA.

5. Open sores or areas of inflammation: This includes acne and also includes the areas around active herpes outbreaks.

6. Suspicious moles, freckles or any spots which have recently changed shape or colour: These should be referred to a medical practitioner as soon as possible.

7. Haemophilia: Bruising in these cases can dangerous.

8. Other clients who bruise very easily: This is a caution rather than a contraindication. There are a lot of blood vessels on the face and even experienced practitioners will hit one from time to time. Around the eyes this can easily lead to the appearance of a black eye. Clients who bruise easily must be aware of this.

9. Inflammation from recent cosmetic procedures: This is especially common for clients who have undergone any form of dermal abrasion. The skin must be fully healed before you proceed.

10. Pacemakers

11. Patients with severe qi deficiency: FCA is generally more dispersing than tonifying. This is due to the number of needles and the need to focus on circulating energy around the face and under wrinkles. It is better not to treat clients with severe qi deficiency particularly if they have been diagnosed with chronic fatigue or an auto immune disease. They tend to feel very flat after treatments and it is not the most appropriate treatment they could be receiving.

12. Patients taking warfarin or other strong blood thinning medications: Due to the very high risk of bruising.

13. Keloid Scars: These are scars that continue to grow throughout their lifetime. They should never be treated with FCA or any other form of skin needling.

This list is not exhaustive and professional judgement is always required.

PRETREATMENT ADVICE FOR THE CLIENT

Listed below are the key points to impart to a potential client when you are taking a FCA booking.

1. Always ask clients not to where any make up to appointments. This is especially important for the first session in which you will be doing more facial diagnosis. In case they do insist on wearing make up make sure you have an area where you can cleanse their skin effectively. If you cannot cleanse their skin properly then hypoallergenic face wipes can be used as an absolute last resort.

2. Ask male clients to shave if they want you to work on the lower half of their face. Generally this part of the face is less affected by the signs of ageing in men due to the exfoliating and circulatory affect of shaving. Beards however make it hard to form a good diagnosis of the face and are harder to needle through.

3. When a client books an appointment it is best to suggest that if they experience any facial herpes they should start taking any regular medication a week before each treatment. Any form of skin penetration triggers the immune system and can lead to an out break of cold sores. Many clients may not have a regular medication but it is still important to provide the warning.

4. For female clients it is better not to schedule treatments premenstrually as the skin can be more sensitive at this time. This can be a difficult issue to raise when taking a first phone booking so is often better explained to existing clients for future appointments.

5. Always explain that there is a small risk of bruising in the area of treatment. This may prompt clients to bring concealer or book appointments on the way home rather than the way out.

6. If you have the knowledge it is a good idea to ask the client about any other cosmetic products they currently use. On inspection you may ask

them to cease using any you feel may work against the treatment. This is especially important for any products that may increase inflammation or dryness such as strong retinol products.

7. It is better to avoid receiving other cosmetic procedures during a course of FCA treatments. Many can cause inflammation that can interfere with the FCA treatment. It is also better if FCA receives the credit for the results it produces and does not receive the blame for any side effects the other treatment causes.

8. Always make sure Clients sign a Patient Consent Form. This should be standard in any modern clinic.

POST TREATMENT PROCEDURE

1. Before the client sits up you can apply an aftercare serum. Organic green tea oil is very effective as it deeply moisturises and protects the skin after treatment (full details of the products we use can be found in the appendix). When applying any products at this stage always wear gloves due to the recent skin penetration. Only massage gently at this stage.

2. Due to the increased blood flow to the head and then subsequent reduction as the needles are removed it is not unusual for clients to feel a little light headed after treatment. Always stay with the client as they sit up.

3. Give the client a glass of water or preferably a warm drink after the treatment to help them wake up. This is particularly important if they are about to drive.

4. Use this time with the client to explain the aftercare procedure. This gives you an excuse to spend a few extra minutes with them and make sure they are feeling okay.

5. Provide a bottle of the green tea oil for clients to use at home between treatments. This protects and nourishes the skin to support the results. They should mix a few drops of oil with a little water in their hands and massage it into their face twice a day.

6. Depending on how you run your clinic you may also ask them to use a jade roller, gua sha or apply another form of cosmetic massage in between treatments.

7. If the instructions you wish your client to follow are particularly complicated it is a good idea to have a prepared document you can give to them. This means you are not reliant on the clients memory which may be a little hazy straight after a treatment. These can also be useful for legal reasons.

Chapter 4

Traditional Chinese Facial Diagnosis

Over the years we have studied with many different schools of Chinese face reading. Some are purely medical in nature. They focus only on how lines or blemishes on the face may reflect deeper pathologies in the individual. Others are far more esoteric predicting the individuals future and reflecting their past.

Here we are only going to focus on aspects of facial diagnosis that will directly improve your ability to achieve great FCA results for your clients.

TCM as it is currently practiced is very consistent in its approach to diagnosis and treatment. There are only small variations between locations. For example the North of China is more focused on cold diseases and the South on warm diseases for obvious geographical reasons.

There have also been slight variations in the focus of TCM as it has left China. In Sydney where I am from for example, many of the Chinese immigrants came from the South of China. Most of my early Professors in fact came from Guang Zhou. Their focus on warm diseases suited the local Sydney climate and so the local TCM practitioners are perhaps better versed in this school of TCM than others.

Despite these minor differences it is surprising how consistent TCM practice is across the world.

It was not always like this. Like Ayuveda in India, TCM knowledge once ran in families. Each family had their own closely guarded secret practices. This would have perhaps continued if it were not for the rise to power of the communist party in 1949. The communist party set about systemising and supporting TCM as the principle system of medicine in the struggling early economy. This more than anything is the reason TCM has been so well documented and is ultimately so consistent throughout China and more recently the rest of the world.

So why are we discussing this in a section on Chinese facial diagnosis? Simple, face reading was not included in this systemisation. Its esoteric roots and claims to be able to predict the future did not sit well with the cultural beliefs of the new rulers of China. Rather than systemise and support face reading it was actively discouraged.

This has meant that most accessible practitioners of TCM face reading now reside outside of China. It has also meant there are larger differences between the various systems. The understanding of the significance of a line in one school is often slightly different to that of another school.

Most of our teachers of facial diagnosis have lived in Chinese communities in Malaysia and Singapore where it is still more openly practiced. In the following section I have elected to focus on the consistencies between the systems and the elements that will be most practical in enhancing your practice of FCA.

They key way in which facial diagnosis can assist FCA is in the recognition of how lines, blemishes and other features on the face may reflect the underlying constitution. This allows us to treat the root cause of the issue through distal points and herbs as well as its manifestation through FCA.

This diagnostic relationship also works in reverse. After many years working with FCA you could take a clients pulse and question them without seeing their face. After making your diagnosis you would most likely be able to predict where the major areas of concern on the face will be.

I mentioned a moment ago that once you can diagnose the underlying constitution or TCM pattern in a client then by treating this you can benefit the appearance of wrinkles on the face. As discussed in the previous section this can be taken one step further. By using FCA to reduce the lines on the face you can improve the health of the underlying organ related to that line.

In many systems of Chinese face reading the face is a little like the ear, palm or sole of the foot. Every area reflects the health of an underlying organ. In auricular acupuncture for example every aspect of the body in TCM can be influenced by a different point. This is the same on the face. Unlike the ear however which is rarely used for diagnosis the face can be used to diagnose issues with the internal organs as well as treat them.

Some teachers take the ability of facial treatments to improve the internal health very seriously. One Feng Shui and face reading teacher we spent time with in Malaysia actually recommended Botox for some of his clients where they were experiencing severe 'suspended swords' (the vertical line between the eyebrows). Botox is a potentially toxic treatment and most acupuncturists will frown upon its use. His belief however was that this line was so detrimental to the health and well being of the client that Botox was the lesser evil.

Facial diagnosis is a huge subject you can study for a lifetime. For our purposes we are going to break it up into two sections with the second section building on the first.

COLOURS OF THE FACE

Understanding what the colours on the face represent is a prerequisite to diagnosing their significance. As is often the case in TCM they are divided into five, one colour to represent each of the five major organs in the body.

Red: Indicates Heat in the body of either deficient or excess origins. This is also the colour of the Heart

Yellow: When the skin is examined closely a yellow colour is far more common than most people think. It usually reflects dampness in the body but can also indicate the presence of heat in some cases. Like the colour this pathology is usually related to the spleen (digestion) in TCM. Jaundice is a more severe example of yellowing of the skin. In most cases the yellow colour we are describing is more subtle and would not be diagnosed as jaundice.

White: Think pale. This is usually related to qi and blood deficiency in TCM and can also represent yang qi deficiency. It is the colour of the lungs but the causes of the paleness can be other organs as well. Do not confuse this paleness with vitiligo or loss of pigmentation in the skin (discussed later) which can have a wider range of causes and will have a clearly delineated border.

Blue/ Black: This is related to kidney deficiency especially kidney yang deficiency but can also be related to cold and/or blood stagnation.

The most common place to see this colour is below the eyes where it represents either kidney deficiency or blood stagnation. It can also be visible around the mouth in rare cases.

Green: This represents a build up of heat and toxins in the body and can also occur in severe cases of dampness. It is often related to the liver.

You will often see clients with a mild green tinge to their entire skin. It is also not uncommon to see it more severely around the mouth where it usually represents a build up of dampness in the spleen.

REGIONS OF THE FACE AND THE SIGNIFICANCE OF LINES AND BLEMISHES IN THESE AREAS

Forehead

The forehead is universally understood to relate to the digestion. In particular the stomach, Spleen, Large Intestine and Small intestine.

Acne is common in this area. If the acne is noticeably more severe in this area it may lead you to focus on damp heat in the intestines as the most likely cause of the acne.

Horizontal lines across the forehead are very common. When you see these you should be focusing on the digestion and the organs mentioned above. In particular consider problems with food absorption and assimilation. This transforming and transporting function is the responsibility of the spleen.

Many systems go so far as to attribute many small lines on the forehead to spleen qi deficiency while one large line alone signifies problems with the Small Intestine.

One exception to this rule is the association of a line along the very top of the forehead with the Urinary Bladder channel.

Moving briefly away from medical Face Reading it is worth noting that in more esoteric schools of face reading three horizontal lines across the forehead are considered fortuitous. This has a close connection with Feng Shui as do many face reading practitioners.

Between the Eyebrows

This area is considered particularly important in Traditional Face Reading. It is often referred to as the 'Seat of the Stamp'. The stamp in China is used as a signature. This expression indicates that the area may to some degree sum up the person. I have read stories that large lines in this area were once cause for exclusion from the courts of the Emperors so seriously was this part of the face taken.

From a FCA perspective this area relates to the liver. Large out breaks of acne almost exclusively in this area indicate the presence of liver fire.

More common in our world is the large vertical line directly between the eyebrows called the 'suspended sword'. It was considered so serious that it may eventually fall down and cut off your foot!

When this line is present you know very quickly where to focus your diagnostic investigations.

Two smaller vertical lines can also be present usually above the border of the nose and the eyes. In different systems these lines can be related to either the spleen or the liver. In practice they often correspond to the pattern of liver attacking spleen but it can vary from client to client. These two lines are considered far less severe than one deep single line in the middle.

Upper Eyelids and Eyebrows

Any drooping or puffiness of the upper eyelids is caused by issues with the spleen and especially spleen qi deficiency. This is very common in older clients and it is important to know how to treat it.

There are multiple different interpretations of the significance of the eyebrows. They range from reflecting the strength of the liver to different sections of the eyebrow reflecting the san jiao, spleen and kidneys respectively.

These theories do not shed much light when diagnosing and are hard to interpret as most women now pluck their eyebrow's. This makes it very easy to get a false read when focusing on the eyebrows alone.

Temples

The area of the temple is related to the gall bladder and the spleen. It is very common to see clusters of acne in this area and if this is the case these are the organs you should focus on, particularly the gall bladder.

The crows feet also run across this area and are also related to the gall bladder and the spleen. Bear in mind that squinting and sun damage play a large role in the formation of these wrinkles. In the Australian countryside it is very common to find these wrinkles are far worse on the right side of clients faces as this is the side of the face exposed to the window's sunlight when driving a car.

Nose

The nose in TCM is controlled by the lungs. Redness around the nostrils and next to the nose is associated with heat and usually wind heat in the lungs. This is especially so if there is peeling or dry skin in the area. Acne in this area is also often associated with lung wind heat.

From there the theories about what the nose reflect tend to differ or at least correspond less between schools. For many schools the tip of the nose represents the heart while for others the spleen. If you see redness in this area think about heat in one of these two organs. A vertical line through the tip of the nose is associated with heart deficiency. This is very hard to treat with FCA and thankfully this treatment is rarely requested.

Horizontal lines across the bridge of the nose can indicate issues with the stomach organ in TCM and can correspond with blood sugar issues such as diabetes.

Some schools also see the nose as a mirror image of the spine with the top representing the neck and the tip the lower back. Blemishes on the nose can therefore be a diagnostic point for wider issues of the spine.

Below the Eyes

Dark marks in this area can indicate either kidney deficiency or blood stagnation. Both potential causes should be investigated and confirmed through other aspects of your diagnosis. In general blood stagnation is a preferable pattern as it is easier to treat.

Swelling and bags under the eyes can also represent issues with the spleen. The most common pattern is phlegm and dampness attacking the spleen with underlying spleen qi deficiency. This results in a failure to lift the qi.

If the bags are softer then dampness is considered predominant over phlegm while if they are firmer then phlegm predominates over dampness. Firmer eye bags related to phlegm are harder to treat and take longer to achieve results.

A line running from the centre of the eye down towards the mouth may indicate issues with the stomach and wrinkles below the outer corner of the eyes are associated with the stomach and large intestine.

Around the Mouth

As a golden rule when you see issues such as discolouration, lack of muscle tone or dryness around the mouth you should think of the digestion and digestive issues.

From there it gets a lot more complicated.

There are theories that divide the lips into 5 different sections related to 5 different organs. In practice these prove very unreliable diagnostic tools especially when dealing with clients of different races and skin tones.

The most important points to note when examining the skin around the mouth are to look for areas or redness or inflammation which are signs of internal heat. In particular look for redness below the mouth indicating heat in the stomach and sometimes directly associated with inflammation of the oesophagus. Be aware that in men redness in these areas can also be the result of having shaved recently.

Look for discolouration particularly signs of yellowness and even green. This is more common than you may think but is hard to pick up without the brightness of a beauticians lamp. This usually indicates dampness.

Make sure the lips are moist. This indicates that the spleen is functioning correctly. Overly moist lips can indicate dampness in the spleen while dryness is a sign of jin Ye (fluid) deficiency.

As a side note for those who are also interested in fertility treatments the depth of the philtrum is associated with fertility. A shallow philtrum or breaks along the philtrum are associated with difficulty in falling pregnant for women.

Cheeks

If there is a lot of inflammation or acne around the acupuncture point Quan Liao (SI 18) look for other signs of heat in the small intestines. This is not one of the primary causes of acne but it can be related.

The area in front of the ears is strongly associated with the liver and gall bladder. It is very common to see isolated patches of acne here and this is a key indicator of heat affecting these organs.

The nasolabial groove running from the corner of the nose to the corner of the mouth generally relates to issues of the gall bladder. Some systems also suggest you should examine more closely the function of the intestines and be wary of constipation exasperating the issue.

The area of the lower cheeks outside the lateral edges of the mouth is associated with the lungs. Acne in this area is often caused by wind heat in the lungs. A vertical line in this area running up outside the line of the mouth indicates issues with the lungs and is very common in smokers.

In some traditional systems this line is also associated with grief. Sadness is of course, the emotion of the lungs.

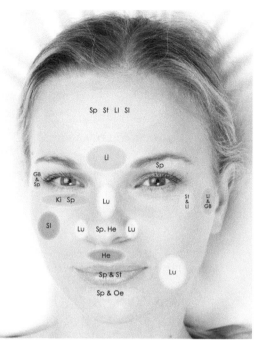

Image 3: Areas of the face and the organs they represent

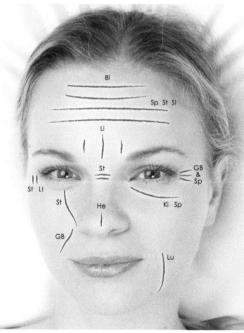

Image 4: Major wrinkles on the face and organs they represent

Chapter 5

Facial Cosmetic Acupuncture Needling Techniques

GUIDING PRINCIPLES OF FCA NEEDLING

These are the basic principles that should be applied wherever possible when employing all the techniques described later

1. Insert distal points first before the facial points and remove the distal points after the facial points.

2. Whenever it is practical needle in an upwards direction. By upwards I mean towards the top of the head. This will assist in lifting the energy and reduce sagging.

3. Use acupuncture points in the area where applicable. If the area you wish to needle is right next to an established acupuncture point use the acupuncture point as your first preference for a stronger treatment.

4. Always plan your treatment so you can access all the points you wish to use. This is shown in the protocols. With so many needles in a small area it is easy to corner yourself so you can't insert the next needle without bumping the existing needles. This causes the client discomfort and potentially dislodges some needles.

5. Always open the sterile packaging of the acupuncture needles in front of the client to reassure them of the sterility of the equipment.

6. If your training and skill allows it, avoid the use of guide tubes wherever possible. The tapping on the guide tube will always jolt a client and make the treatment less comfortable and relaxing. We realise more and more of our students are only trained with guide tubes but it is amazing how quickly most adapt especially when using short high quality needles.

7. Ask the client to shut their eyes if applying any pretreatment alcohol. The fumes from the alcohol can sting their eyes. The requirement to use swabs vary based on location but alcohol is dehydrating and best avoided on the face where possible.

8. Always ask the client to close their eyes during FCA treatments. Many clients are nervous about needles. Even when done painlessly the sight of acupuncture needles up close to their their eyes will be disconcerting.

9. Always count the number of needles you insert. Clients will twitch and move when they are on the table and shallow needles can slip out. It is important to be sure you have them all and that the client does not find one down the front of their clothes later in the day.

10. Use cotton pads rather than cotton wool balls to withdraw the needles. They are more absorptive and don't leave bits of cotton on the face especially on beards.

11. When withdrawing the needles hold pressure on the points for several seconds. Around the eyes or if you suspect bruising hold the pressure for at least 30 seconds as bruising in this areas can be more severe.

TYPES OF NEEDLES

FCA is best performed with 15mm, plastic handled needles. Originally we only used 16 gauge needles but as gauges have reduced we have introduced 12 gauge needles as well as an alternative for particularly sensitive clients. Overall the stimulation of the slightly thicker needles produces better results. If high quality needles are used with good technique there is little difference in sensation for the client.

Always purchase plastic handled needles rather than metal handles as they weigh less. Many of the needles are inserted very superficially and can fall out if the client moves a lot over the 28 minutes. This is made worse by the extra weight in metal handles.

Spend a little more and buy good quality needles as you are placing a lot of needles into very sensitive skin. When purchasing your longer needles for distal points I recommend sticking to this quality policy. You will only be using a handful and it is better if the whole treatment is as relaxing as possible.

Finally gold needles are sometimes recommended for tonifying the skin in traditional approaches. In clinic there is no major improvement in results when using these needles. Generally the quality of the gold needles is lower than high quality stainless steel needles you can now purchase.

NEEDLE RETENTION TIMES

In theory acupuncture needles should be retained for 28 minutes. In the ancient theories this is the amount of time it takes the qi to do one full circuit of the body. In general practice we may shorten or elongate this time based on the constitution of the client and based on the goals we are trying to achieve.

FCA can present a particular challenge in this respect as it can take a lot longer to insert all the needles than in a normal acupuncture session. This means that in more intricate cases up to 10 minutes may have elapsed between the insertion of the first needle and the last. At which point then do you start your 28 minutes?

In general as FCA is quite a dispersing treatment it is better to err on the side of caution. It is better to time from the first insertion than from the last. This is especially true of the first treatment when you are not yet sure how the client will feel afterwards.

There is an element of judgement that needs to be applied here. You want the maximum treatment time to achieve the best possible results but never at the expense of the health of the client. Be particularly careful to use the shorter treatment times when dealing with older or weaker clients.

Always bear in mind that you will need to check the clock as you start inserting the needles rather than glancing upwards on your way out of the room.

THREADING

Threading techniques are the bread and butter of most FCA protocols. Put very simply threading involves inserting multiple acupuncture needles under a wrinkle or scar.

The aim of the technique is too act a little like subscision which was explained earlier. The needles are inserted 1-2mm from the border of the wrinkle you wish to reduce and then 'threaded' under the wrinkle. The aim is that the needle finishes or at least passes through the border between the bottom of the wrinkle and the healthy tissue below.

It should be noted that some teachers advocate inserting straight through the wrinkle. This technique is also effective but is less comfortable for the client and often less practical with deep wrinkles.

Needling depth and angle are important and will vary based on the severity of the wrinkle and the elasticity of the clients skin. Many practitioners like to insert needles only on one side of the wrinkle while others like to insert from both sides to ensure ample coverage of the base of the wrinkle.

In an ideal world where possible the needles will be directed upward (toward the top of the head rather than the chin) to lift the skin and this is done where possible. In reality practical considerations often determine the direction of the needles.

For example if you are planning to insert needles under the 3 horizontal lines on the forehead of a client, you must plan to only insert needles from one side as otherwise the needles from the previous wrinkle will interfere with the future insertions.

It is important to note that when wrinkles are treated this way they will often 'stand up' and clients may comment that they look raised and worse immediately after treatment. This is a good sign that you have engaged the healing process and will achieve good results.

Threading techniques can be used on any wrinkle or long scar. They are most commonly employed on horizontal lines across the forehead, frown lines, nasolabilial lines, vertical lip lines and marionette lines.

SUBCISION

Subcision is very similar to the threading technique but requires a separate explanation as it is usually employed in a circular way around scars. In this way it is identical to what was called 'circling the dragon' in the ancient texts.

The needles are inserted from 1-2mm outside the border of the scar with the intention of needling directly under the scar. The needle should finish or pass through the border between the scar and the healthy tissue below.

When done well on depressed (hypotrophic) scars it will look like the scar 'pops up'. This noticeably decreases the appearance of the scar. With smaller depressed acne scars one needle may be used per scar as there is not always sufficient space for multiple needles.

LIFTING AND PINNING

The theory behind this technique draws from some of the ancient needle manipulations to tonify acupuncture points. In these practices the needle is inserted and then twirled rapidly. The tissue becomes entwined around the needle. Done correctly this temporarily binds the tissue to the needle. It can feel like the needle is stuck and harder to withdraw.

To apply this in FCA you use your other hand to lift the skin upwards and outwards. Once the skin is in the position you want you insert the needle. The needle is inserted through the raised skin into the skin below. The needle is then twirled rapidly. The aim is to bind the tissue around the needle so pinning the skin into this raised position.

A good example of the use of this technique is in sagging cheeks. The point of insertion is St 3. First the other hand is used to pull the skin from St 3 up towards the outer corner of the eye. The skin may move between 1-2cm. By pulling the skin upwards in this way you have very slightly folded the skin. This means that the skin you have pulled up is now in contact with skin that was higher on the face.

Once it is in the correct position insert the needle into the point St 3. Please note that we are referring to the skin that was originally in the position of St 3. It will now be raised slightly and will no longer line up with the lower border of the nose. Insert towards the outer corner of the eye. Needle through St 3 into the higher skin it is now in contact with. Twirl the needle rapidly and try to bind the skin in this position.

Essentially you are trying to lift and stretch the skin upwards and outwards and then 'pin' it into this position. When done properly it is a subtle but effective technique.

It is most commonly used to stretch out nasolabial lines and lift the skin on the cheeks but can be employed elsewhere on the face as well.

INTRADERMAL ACUPUNCTURE NEEDLES

Intradermal acupuncture needles are small 3-6mm long needles usually with a small 1.5mm diameter wring on the end. They range in gauge from 0.12 to 0.14.

There are whole schools of FCA who only use intradermal needles for all their treatments.

The key advantage of intradermal needles is their ability to be taped in place and left in the client's skin over night. This provides a very long lasting and effective treatment which is not available with conventional acupuncture needles.

Unfortunately the key advantage is also the major potential pitfall. By leaving the needles in overnight you run the risk of the client knocking them out. The tiny needles may then be swallowed or enter another orifice on the clients face.

If using intradermals you should also check your insurance that you are covered to leave the needles in overnight as this varies based on location.

If you are able to and feel confident to employ intradermals then they can be extremely useful and an extra weapon in your armoury against stubborn wrinkles.

They are most commonly used to thread under and through wrinkles. Due to their length they are more often inserted directly into the wrinkle than to the side of the wrinkle. The needles must be inserted almost completely parallel to the skin so the wring on the end can sit flat to the skin and be taped down effectively.

Make sure to use the correct tape to hold the needles down and apply it very carefully. Clients must be given instructions not to touch the tape and will have to avoid washing their face overnight. It is usually best to do these treatments last thing in the evening and remove them the next morning but this can also be done in reverse. This means you need to book two appointments and this treatment must be planned in advance.

Always count the number of intradermal needles you insert to ensure they are all there the next day.

These treatments are now less used due to the risk and potential liability involved. If you are able to use them they are particularly effective against multiple vertical lip lines with one intradermal per wrinkle.

ACUPUNCTURE POINTS AND ASHI POINTS

If you are going to needle a particular area as part of the treatment it makes sense to make use of any local acupuncture points as part of this process. Unlike other cosmetic treatments we are always seeking to improve the client's constitution as part of every treatment. The use of both known acupuncture points and ashi points assists in this endeavour.

When needling acupuncture points wherever possible needle upwards. The lifting and pinning technique described earlier can also be employed on many of these points to further lift the skin.

LIP ENHANCEMENT

This is not actually a needling technique on its own but a specific application of acupuncture needles to enhance the lips.

This is done by taking 3-4 acupuncture needles and holding them together parallel in the finger tips. The tips of the needles must be at the same length.

The needles are then rapidly inserted and withdrawn along the border of the lips. It should take several minutes of constant repeated insertion to cover the border all the way around the lips.

This technique creates swelling in the lips that mimics the appearance of collagen injections. The swelling will usually reach its peak after about 30 minutes and will last several days.

This can be performed before special events like weddings. Bruising is very rare with this technique due to the needle location and shallow depth of penetration.

Although not strictly health enhancing unlike the rest of the techniques in this book it is impressive and allows many clients who want this look to avoid injectables.

In beauty clinics a very similar technique is sometimes performed with micro needle rollers. I now prefer to perform lip enhancement this way as it is less uncomfortable for the client and quicker to perform.

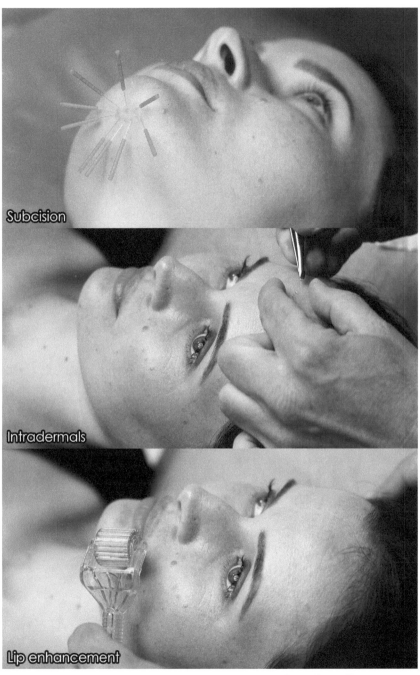

Subcision

Intradermals

Lip enhancement

Image 5: i) Subcision around a scar ii) Inserting intradermal needles iii) Using a micro needle roller to perform lip enhancement

DISTAL POINTS

Distal Points in FCA are essentially any acupuncture point not located on the face or neck. They should always be inserted according to the underlying TCM pattern presenting in each client. This is discussed in more detail later but assisting the wider health of the client is the prime reason for using distal points.

The other key reason to use distal points is to keep the person 'grounded' and stop too much blood (and qi) rushing to their head. For this reason the best distal points are usually located in the feet where possible.

Common distal points for those who are not able to differentiate TCM patterns are Tai Chong (Liv 3), Nei Ting (St 44), Zu Ling Qi (GB 43), Shen Mai (Bl 62), Zhao Hai (K 6). These points can be used in rotation.

Always place the needles in the client's feet before the FCA needles and take them out after you have taken out the FCA needles.

THE INFLUENCE OF SKIN COLOUR ON NEEDLING DEPTH

This question arises far more often than you might think. The most common question is usually from clients with darker skin who ask "will shallow needling work as well for me as I have thicker skin?" This and other questions are becoming more common as first the make up industry, and now the beauty industry, customise beauty treatments for darker skin tones.

In the beauty industry this was largely prompted by some cosmetic treatments permanently damaging their clients melanin producing cells. Many clients with darker skin permanently lost pigmentation and were left with white patches. The most common culprit was deep dermal abrasion. If you attend a cosmetic expo now it is very common to see caveats on products that they are safe for black skin.

Darker skin is also far more likely to suffer from keloid scars, a type of scar which continues to grow throughout its lifetime. These should never be treated as you can potentially increase the speed of their growth.

Thankfully skin colour makes no difference to the effectiveness of FCA treatments. In fact there is very little difference in the skin thickness for clients of all different skin tones. On average the epidermis is between 0.1 - 0.15mm thick and the dermis below this is between 1.35-1.4mm thick.

As you can see the difference is only fractions of a millimetre. Any differences in facial shape for darker skin sometimes ascribed to having 'thicker skin' are actually caused by thicker underlying connective tissue rather than thicker skin.

From an acupuncturists point of view thicker underlying connective tissue may allow you to penetrate slightly deeper if you wish to but in most cases you are aiming for the border of the wrinkle/scar with the healthy underlying tissue so it makes very little difference to the treatment.

Chapter 6

Chinese Medicine Pattern Differentiation and Constitutional Treatment

Below we will discuss some of the main facial issues clients present with. In each case we will go through the major TCM patterns that may cause the issue. We will then describe the needling techniques, distal points and internal herbal medicine which is appropriate.

I am aware in writing this that the types of training received by acupuncturists differ greatly. If you are not trained in herbal medicine or traditional Chinese diagnosis this is not a problem. The prescriptions for the localised needling will still work very well for you. For those who are traditionally trained the supporting treatments are a huge bonus. It is something that differentiates FCA from most mainstream cosmetic practices.

There is also an added a section on Chinese Herbal medicine preparation for external use in the appendix. It covers important external formulas that can be prepared in your clinic based on your diagnosis.

WRINKLES

GENERAL PRINCIPLES FOR WRINKLE TREATMENTS

Needle under either end of the wrinkle to begin shortening it. This is a common technique to help prevent the wrinkle elongating.

Thread multiple needles under the wrinkle all the way long its length. In many cases the wrinkle will actually lift up during and after the treatment. This may worry the client temporarily but it is actually a good sign that the minor inflammation required to begin the healing process is taking place.

Specific techniques for each different type of wrinkle are explained in the step by step techniques for facial issues later in the book.

TCM PATTERN DIFFERENTIATION AND CONSTITUTIONAL TREATMENT OF WRINKLES

a) Liver and Kidney Yin Deficiency or Jing Deficiency

This is the most common cause of wrinkles on the face. Unfortunately being related to the kidneys it also the most difficult to treat.

The wrinkles in this case tend to be deeper and more set in than wrinkles caused by qi and blood deficiency. This is to be expected as as the kidney energy and jing fade throughout our lives meaning this type of wrinkles will be more common in older clients.

In clinic you will also see women experiencing menopause who will fit into this category. They often display yin deficient heat patterns leading too hot flushes.

Common Distal Points

Tai Xi (K 3), Guan Yuan (Ren 4), Qi Hai (Ren 6), Tai Chong (Liv 3), San Yin Jiao (Sp 6)

Internal Herbal Medicine

Internal medicine is important for this group especially if there are other diagnostic factors pointing towards kidney deficiency. For herbal medicine to be effective it will usually have to be taken long term.

Common Formulas include

- Kidney yin deficiency: Liu Wei Di Huang wan or Zuo Gui Yin.
- Kidney and liver yin deficiency: Qi Ju Di Huang Wan or Er Zhi Wan.
- Jing deficiency: Use the above formulas or You Gui Wan

b) Qi and Blood Deficiency with Predominant Heart Blood Deficiency

These are usually thin shallow wrinkles accompanied by pale and lustreless skin. This is the key differentiation between these and the deeper wrinkles seen in kidney deficiency. Many clients of course may have a combination of both.

Common Distal Points

Zu San Li (St 36), Xue Hai (Sp10), Zhong Wan (Ren 12), Ju Que (Ren 14)

Internal Medicine

The principle formula for this pattern is Gui Pi Wan. It is excellent at tonifying the heart blood and with the high does of Huang Qi it guides the energy upwards towards the head. Alternatives include Ba Zhen Wan or Bu Zhong Yi Qi Wan if there is more qi deficiency.

c) Qi and Blood Stagnation Particularly Related to the Liver

This pattern refers to wrinkles in specific locations such as frown lines between the eyebrows.

Common Distal Points

Tai Chong (Liv 3), Nei Guan (P 6), Yang Ling Quan (GB 34)

Internal Medicine

The formula used depends on the severity of the liver qi stagnation. The most common formula is Jia Wei Xiao Yao Wan. This is perhaps the most commonly used formula in the Western world due to the high stress levels prevalent in every day life. If there is co-existing blood stagnation then use Tong Qiao Huo Xue Wan, Tao Hong Si Wu Wan or Xue Fu Zhu Yu Wan.

SAGGING SKIN

GENERAL PRINCIPLES FOR TREATING SAGGING SKIN

This most commonly occurs in specific locations such as under the eyes, along the jowls, chin and down on the neck. Around the eyes it is commonly seen concurrently with puffiness. The key principal of treatment is lifting the skin.

Specific needling techniques for each area will be described in the Step by Step Instructions for each cosmetic issue.

TCM PATTERN DIFFERENTIATION AND CONSTITUTIONAL TREATMENT OF SAGGING SKIN

a) Spleen Qi Deficiency

The key pattern here is that weakness of the spleen qi, fails to lift the qi, leading to sagging.

In many cases the pattern may be combined with kidney deficiency which must be dealt with simultaneously.

Common Distal Points

Zu San Li (St 36), San Yin Jiao (Sp 6), Yin Ling Quan (Sp 9), Bai Hui (Ren 20), Zhong Wan (Ren 12)

Internal Herbal Medicine

The number one formula for lifting qi is Bu Zhong Yi Qi Wan. If the client is suffering a lot of dampness Xiang Sha Liu Jun Zi Wan or Shen Ling Bai Zhu Wan can be used or Bu Zhong Yi Qi San can be combined with Ping Wei Wan or Huo Xiang Zheng Qi Wan.

SCARS

GENERAL PRINCIPLES FOR TREATING SCARS

Scars are more obviously attributable to external causes than many of the other facial issues. In FCA the most common scars you will see are acne scars followed by scars from traumatic injuries. The principals of treatment are similar and depend more on the shape and location of the scar than any underlying TCM pattern.

From a TCM perspective scars are generally considered to be caused by qi and blood stagnation. Their location is considered particularly important as they may cut across important channels and and so affect the underlying health of the body. This is particularly true of scarring due to gynaecological procedures.

These scars often cut across a lot of important meridians leading to further health complications. They can be treated in the same way as facial scars.

When treating acne scars one difficulty can be the continuing presence of acne outbreaks. Keep in mind you must not needle into areas of inflammation such as acne and this can interfere with the treatment. In these cases it is often better to pause and try to deal with the acne itself and prevent further scarring before addressing the existing scars.

Circular Scars

These are best treated using the technique traditionally called 'circling the dragon' or subcision.

The process has been discussed earlier and involves needling underneath the scar from multiple different directions. The idea is to get underneath the scar to cause minor trauma in the area where the scar connects to the healthy tissue below. This process helps cause a separation between the scar and the underlying tissue. The micro-trauma then helps create a new layer of collagen and elastin in the area.

This technique can be used on all types of scars but is especially useful on hypotrophic (depressed scars) as creating this separation under the scar can help the depressed scar 'pop up'.

This technique is particularly useful in FCA as most acne scars are hypotrophic scars. It works best on the larger scars.

When there are multiple very small scars, like icepick scars caused by blackheads or large areas of burn scars it is often best to combine the treatment with a micro-needle roller. The roller can cover these wider areas and you can then reserve the acupuncture needles for the larger scars. This avoids literally having to insert hundreds of needles in each session. A traditional dermal hammer or seven star needle can also be used but most patients report less discomfort with a micro-needle roller.

For many patients I have treated with burn scars, acupuncture was not an option as the acupuncture needles would only have been around the edge and missed the large centre of the burns. This is especially true of patients with burns over 5cm across usually from fires and oil or water burns.

Micro-needling can pass over the entire area of the scar far less painfully than acupuncture needles. What is often not understood about the wound healing cascade is that as part of the process collegenease is released. This is an enzyme that breaks down old misaligned collagen fibres to allow a new smooth matrix of collagen to form.

In scars collagen fibres usually line up parallel rather than in a smooth cross section. This causes the appearance of the scar. By creating such a high number of punctures, micro-needling dramatically induces this wound healing cascade which can break down large patches of scar tissue and produce smoother flatter skin.

If the scars are fairly fresh or particularly extensive it is always worth considering whether you feel qualified to assist this condition or should it be referred to a medical practitioner.

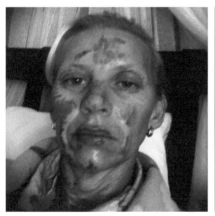 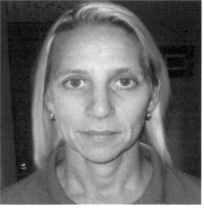

Before   After

Image 6: Images of a client who received severe burns from an Australian grass fire. The first photo is taken while she was still in hospital. As she was an existing client we were able to start her on a a course of micro-needling as soon as all the scabs had fallen off . She then continued with weekly treatment for 3 months. The after photo is taken at the end of the 3 months. In this case the before and after photos were taken by the client herself and are used with her permission.

LONG THIN SCARS

I mention these separately as they are the second most common type of scar on the face and are usually due to traumatic injury. The principles are essentially the same as those you use to treat long thin wrinkles. Place a needle at either end of the scar pointing towards the scar. Then thread needles underneath the scar along its borders. The depth of penetration will vary depending on the size of the scar.

Common Distal Points

Distal Points in scarring should be applied on the basis of any underlying health pattern observed. If in doubt a few points should alway be placed in the feet to draw excessive blood flow away from the head.

Internal Herbal Medicine

This depends very much on the differential diagnosis which is often more disparate in scars from external causes. The general principle is to circulate the blood where appropriate. Formulas, which can be used, include Xue Fu Zhu Yu Wan or Tao Hong Si Wu Wan or the patent medicine Yunnan Pai Yao.

ACNE
GENERAL PRINCIPLES FOR ASSISTING ACNE

Acne is often neglected in teachings about FCA. The problem with this is that in the majority of clients with acne scarring there will be some continuing acne. Knowing how to assist acne will allow you to better assist their acne scars.

Acne presents a challenge for a FCA practitioner. The extent of the acne coverage will largely dictate whether you can needle the face at all. It is always contraindicated to needle directly into pustules or areas of inflammation which can limit your options. Great care must be taken to limit contact with the skin so as to limit the spread of bacteria.

Treatment usually involves a fine balance of distal acupuncture points combined with limited FCA on the healthy skin surrounding the acne out breaks.

Dermal hammers or micro-needling can be employed over areas of black heads with little inflammation. These effectively increase blood flow assisting detoxification in these areas.

More than all the other conditions mentioned so far effective treatment of acne involves good diagnosis of the underlying TCM pattern. This can be combined with the use of herbal medicines and dietary advice. As internal herbal medicine is so important for this group I have listed some prescription formulas that are very effective in addition to the pre-formulated patent medicine.

In all cases of acne, it is important to ensure that the client is making regular bowel movements. Constipation will contribute to the build up of heat in the body leading to more acne. For many women it is also important to address any menstrual or gynaecological issues as these may be contributing to the acne outbreaks.

Remember the location of acne points can be a useful diagnostic tool. Outbreaks of acne occurring on specific acupuncture points can indicate the presence of heat in particular acupuncture meridians. This is particularly important if the acne occurs symmetrically on the same acupuncture point on both sides of the face. This reduces the chances that the location is coincidental.

Where the acne is darker in colour consider the possibility of blood stagnation co-existing with the heat in the system and modify the treatment accordingly.

In addition to the distal points listed in the pattern prescriptions some distal acupuncture points are especially useful for acne in particular locations. These include

Forehead – Nei Ting (St 44)

In Front of ears – Xing Jian (Liv 2), Li Gou (Liv 5)

Above the mouth – Yin Xi (He 6)

Acne generally takes longer to treat. A course of treatment is rarely less than 3 to 6 months but clients may begin to see results after only 1 to 2 sessions.

TCM PATTERN DIFFERENTIATION AND CONSTITUTIONAL TREATMENT OF ACNE

a) Wind Heat in the Lungs

The skin is generally red and the acne lesions are generally papules though there may still be some pustules.

Common Distal Points

He Gu (LI 4), Qu Chi (LI 11), Pian Li (LI 6), Xue Hai (Sp 10), Chi Ze (Lu 5)

Internal Herbal Medicine

The best formula is Pi Pa Qing Fei Yin (Pi Pa Ye, Gan Cao, Ren Shen, Huang Lian Huang Bai, Sang Bai Pi) and add Yu Xing Cao. This is not normally available as pills or a patent. The best patent normally available is often Qing Qi Hua Tan Wan.

b) Damp Heat in the Spleen and Stomach

The key differentiating factor is that the facial skin is usually oily whereas it is often dry in cases of wind heat. The lesions are also more likely to be pustules though papules can also be present. Constipation is more likely to be present in this pattern and must be treated as part of any effective treatment.

Common Distal Points

Shang Ju Xu (St 37), Xia Ju Xu (St 39), Zhi Gou (SJ 6), Da Heng (Sp 15)

The points listed for the wind heat pattern can also be used simultaneously.

Internal Herbal Medicine

As a prescription use Yin Chen Hao Tang and add Ku Shen and Jin Yin Hua

This is a purging formula so it should only be used on strong clients with excess heat.

c) Disorder of Chong and Ren (Liver Qi Stagnation)

They key diagnostic point is that the acne occurs at specific times in the menstrual cycle. Any issues with the menstrual cycle must be addressed as a preliminary step in an effective treatment.

Common Distal Points

Tai Chong (Liv 3), San Yin Jiao (Sp 6)

Internal Herbal Medicine

This depends a lot on the individual differentiation. A common prescription would be to use Xiao Yao Tang and add Mu Dan Pi, Hong Hua, Sheng Di and Yi Mu Cao. Patent formulas such as Xiao Yao Wan or Jia Wei Xiao Yao Wan are often very useful in these cases.

VITILIGO

This is a loss of localised pigmentation resulting in white spots or patches. It usually occurs on darker skin tones but can occur on lighter skin. It is differentiated by a demarcated border with the surrounding skin.

I have put out several videos on assisting vitiligo with micro-needing in the past as this can in some cases be very effective. FCA alone will rarely produce results and I mainly included it in this book so practitioners know how to proceed when dealing with their first case.

Vitiligo is often secondary to other serious underlying medical conditions or may occur in isolation. It is vey important to do a thorough assessment of the clients health before preceding with any treatments. It is best to explain and be honest that the treatment is unlikely to produce major results and then ask them if they want to proceed. If you do proceed with treatment always do a test patch and then wait a few weeks before continuing with further treatment.

In TCM vitiligo is usually caused by qi and blood deficiency with wind attack. It needs to be treated on a case by case basis with both local and distal points. Both internal herbal medicine and external herbal medicine are useful in these cases. Please see the appendix on external herbal medicine for appropriate preparations.

Internal Herbal Treatment

Use Shou Wu Yin (He Shou Wu, Chi Shao, Bai Shao, He Huan Pi, Hong Hua, Yuan Zhi, Xia Gu Cao, Dang Gui, Sheng Di, Shu Di, Dan Shen, Long Dan Cao, Hei Zhi Ma) and combine with Fang Feng Tang (Fang Feng, Di Gu Pi, Zhi Zi, Wang Bu Liu Xing, Jing Jie, Zhi Shi, Dang Shen, Sheng Di, Gan Cao).

Chapter 7

Step by Step Instructions for Specific Cosmetic Issues

Below are detailed step by step instructions for treating the major issues you will be confronted with in clinic. The instructions have been designed as they make use of all the needling techniques described in the book. Once you are familiar with all these techniques you can combine them with the other principles described in this book to innovate and effectively treat any combination of skin type and issues your clients may present with.

SAGGING NECK AND NECK LINES

1. Needle Yi Feng (SJ 17).

2. Needle Tian Rong (SI 17) upwards towards Tongue.

3. Needle Lian Quan (Ren 23) directly upwards to lift the area.

4. Needle horizontally with multiple needles from the chin downwards to above the clavicle depending on how low the sagging goes. This should only be done on loose skin where the skin can be effectively lifted away from the wind pipe and the needles inserted parallel to the skin. After lifting the skin take care when releasing it that the needles sit down gently. The needles should be inserted about 4-5mm in depth (parallel) to ensure they stay in place. Never insert needles perpendicularly in this area! This technique can be used directly on lines in the area as a threading technique.

5. When treating the neck always be aware of the location of the carotid artery and the wind pipe. Caution should always be taken when needling in this area.

6. Combine this treatment with the sagging cheeks protocol listed below to increase the benefit to the sagging neck.

MARIONETTE LINES (VERTICAL LINES FROM THE CHIN TO THE CORNER OF THE MOUTH)

1. Employ threading along the line starting at either end but making sure all the needles point in an upward direction.

2. The number of needles used will depend on the length of the line.

MOUTH FROWN LINES (VERTICAL LINES NEXT TO THE MOUTH)

1. Needle Ju Liao (St 3) and Quan Liao (SI 18) upwards and towards the top of the ear using the lifting and pinning technique.

2. Then thread along the line with the needles pointing upwards. Make sure there is needle at the bottom of the line to shorten it. Ideally use points such as Di Cang (St 4) if they are on the line.

3. In practice this line usually forms part of the marionette lines and nasolabial folds and is needled as part of this treatment.

NASOLABIAL FOLDS (THE CORNER OF THE NOSE TO THE CORNER OF THE MOUTH)

1. Needle Ju Liao (St 3) and Quan Liao (SI 18) upwards and towards the top of the ear using the lifting and pinning technique to stretch the skin.

2. Insert a needle at the start of the line close to Ying Xiang (LI 20) and then thread along the line with each needle pointing in an upwards direction.

3. When you reach the end of the line make sure you place a needle under the end of the line.

4. Needle the point Di Cang (St 4) if it crosses this line.

SAGGING CHEEKS

1. Use the points Jia Che (St 6) and Da Ying (St 5). Needle both of these points in an upwards direction using the lifting and pinning technique. Extra ashi points can also be used along the jaw line with this lifting and pining technique to reduce sagging of the jaw line. These will all be needled in an upward direction.

2. Needle Extra Points Jia Cheng Jiang in an upwards direction. Do not try to lift and pin here due to the lack of tissue.

3. Needle Quan Liao (SI 18) in an upwards and outwards direction towards the top of the ear. Use the lifting and pinning technique.

4. You can also use extra ashi points in the immediate area to help pull the skin upwards and outwards. This technique is also useful to start stretching out the nasolabial lines.

5. Needle Ting Gong (SI 19) as a supportive point. It is a key lymphatic drainage point in cosmetic massage to drain excess fluids from the face. Excessive fluid is common in conjunction with facial sagging.

VERTICAL LIP LINES (VERTICAL LINES ABOVE AND BELOW THE MOUTH)

1. These can be treated either with traditional needles or benefit greatly from the use of intradermals.

2. Needle Ju Liao (St 3) upwards and towards the top of the ear using the lifting and pinning technique to stretch the skin.

3. Insert one needle into each line or as many as possible depending on the density of wrinkles.

4. Needle in an upwards direction both above and below the mouth. If needling both above and below the mouth needle above the mouth first to allow access to insert the needles below the mouth afterwards.

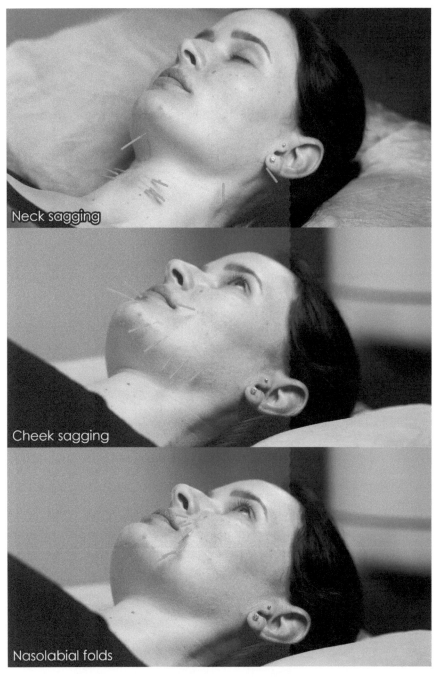

Neck sagging

Cheek sagging

Nasolabial folds

Image 7: i) Sagging Neck Treatment ii) Sagging Cheeks iii) Nasolabial Lines combined with Marionette Lines

HORIZONTAL LINES BELOW THE EYE

1.   Thread needles along the line. Start closest to the nose and needle from below the line very slightly upwards under the wrinkle(s). Only needle shallowly and avoid manipulation to avoid bruising. Placing the other hand on the lower foramen of the eye can help ensure you do not needle too close to the eye.

2.   Place a final needle under the end of the wrinkle to shorten it.

3.   Needle Si Bai (ST 2) in an upwards direction towards the eye. Do not needle too deeply and do not employ any manipulation to avoid bruising.

4.   Keep the pressure on these points for 30 seconds after withdrawing the needles to avoid bruising.

5.   It is better to avoid needling this area within 48 hours of a special evening in case of bruising. If you have one a very low power laser acupuncture kit is very useful to treat below the eyes before special events. Beneficial points include Cheng Qi (St 1), Jing Ming (Bl 1), Qiu Hou (extra) and Tong Zi Liao (GB 1).

BAGS BELOW THE EYES

1.   Find the lower border of the eye bag and thread needles along the line. Start closest to the nose and needle from below the line very slightly upwards under the border. Only needle shallowly and avoid manipulation to avoid bruising. Placing the other hand on the lower foramen of the eye can help ensure you do not needle too close to the eye.

2.   Needle Si Bai (ST 2) in an upwards direction towards the eye. Do not needle too deeply and do not employ any manipulation to avoid bruising.

3.   Keep the pressure on these points for 30 seconds after withdrawing the needles to avoid bruising.

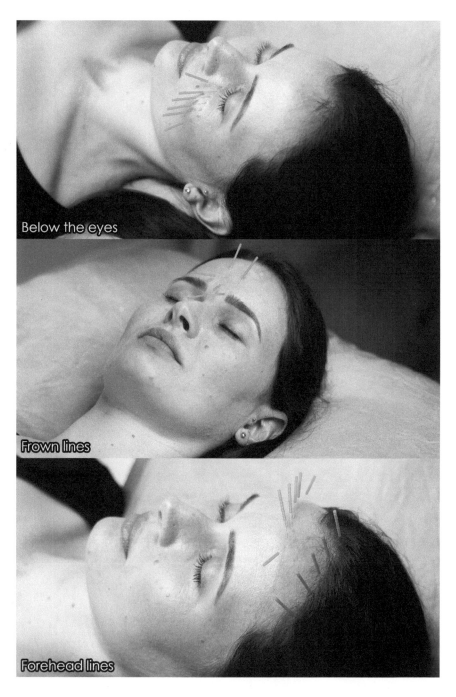

Below the eyes

Frown lines

Forehead lines

Image 8: i) Lines Below the Eyes ii) Frown Lines iii) Forehead Lines

CROW'S FEET

1. Thread one needle under the end of each wrinkle and if the wrinkle is long enough insert a second needle further along the wrinkle in a slightly upwards direction.

2. An alternative treatment is to take a 30mm (1 cun) needle and needle below the entire Tai Yang area in an upwards direction. This needle must be threaded carefully and will pass below all crows feet wrinkles.

3. Again there is a high risk of bruising in this area so be careful before special events.

HORIZONTAL LINES ON THE BRIDGE OF THE NOSE

1. Insert one needle into either end of the line or as close as possible.

2. A third needle can be threaded from below the line if there is enough space.

FROWN LINES (VERTICAL LINES BETWEEN THE EYEBROWS)

1. If there is only one large line in the centre (Suspended Sword) then needle into either end of line from above and below and thread further needles under it in an upwards direction if there is space.

2. If there are several smaller lines then place one needle under the lower end of each in an upwards direction. A further needle can be place at the higher end of the wrinkle pointing downwards if there is space.

DROOPING EYELIDS

1. Needle the points Zan Zhu (BL 2), You Yao (extra) and Si Zhu Kong (SJ 23) in an upwards direction to start to lift the skin in the area.

FOREHEAD LINES (HORIZONTAL LINES ACROSS THE FOREHEAD)

1. To lift the forehead upwards and help stretch out these lines needle Shen Ting (DU 24) in an upwards direction and then you can place several needles along a line jsut inside the hair line. Each point should be needled upwards to life and stretch the skin of the forehead. Acupuncture points you can use in this area include Mei Chong (BL 3), Qu Chai (BL 4), Tou Lin Qi (GB 15), Ben Shen (GB 13) and Tou Wei (ST 8). All are located 0.5 chun within the hair line forming a convenient line for lifting the skin of the forehead.

2. Needle into the end of each line and then thread along the course of the wrinkle. Ideally threading should be from below the wrinkle in an upwards direction.

3. If there are multiple wrinkles in the area you may want to focus on one and thread along this one and only needle the ends of the other wrinkles.

4. Do not needle too deeply on the forehead as it can be a sensitive area. In fact surprisingly many clients find the forehead the most painful part of the face for FCA.

Chapter 8

Complementary Treatments

WHY USE COMPLEMENTARY TREATMENTS?

A.   They can improve results. This is the no 1 and most important reason as that is what the treatments are all about.

B.   They can relax the client. It is worth remembering that needles are the second biggest phobia in the Western world. A short massage before a treatment can help the client relax. When the client is relaxed and some of the tension has left their face those with needle phobias experience the treatments as less traumatic.

C.   They allow you time to more accurately assess the clients skin prior to commencing treatment. Any form of massage performed prior to FCA allows you to assess the client's skin in a less invasive way than staring at them through a beauticians lamp. This improved assessment of their skin will improve your treatments.

D.   They allow you more flexibility to create unique custom treatments packages designed to suit your clients needs.

WHEN TO USE COMPLEMENTARY TREATMENTS?

It is important to remember that any form of massage needs to be performed prior to the FCA treatment. Some of the reasons for this I have listed above. Additionally after FCA the skin has to be treated as though it has gone through an invasive procedure. This means any massage equipment such as Jade Rollers, Gua Shas or Cups that are applied immediately after FCA have to be treated as though they have been exposed to blood. They should never again be used on other clients.

The products can be disinfected but they cannot be sterilised easily and the practitioner is exposing their clients to a hygiene risk and themselves to a legal and moral risk.

Please note the difference between the terms disinfect and sterilise. Disinfection can be performed with alcohol, detergents or a UV sanitiser. It kills bacteria but does not kill blood born diseases. Sterilisation does kill known blood born diseases. It is most commonly performed using gamma ray radiation or ethylene oxide in laboratory conditions. Formerly many acupuncturists used to sterilise acupuncture needles using an autoclaving machine. This kills blood born diseases but is not economical in most modern clinics.

There is some debate as to whether Jade Rollers, Gua Shas and Cups can be reused on the same client after disinfection. This is common with many products including micro-needle rollers in modern beauty clinics. In this system the client's name is written on the product or its casing. It can then be reopened for their next visit. Unfortunately this system is very vulnerable to human error and is not recommended.

Another option is to allow the client to take the Jade Roller or other complementary product home with them in between treatments. This depends on how comfortable you feel with this and how you choose to run your clinic.

It is tempting to find ways to use tools like jade rollers after skin needling treatments to 'cool the skin and close the pores' but there are risks involved however you organise it. Overall it is much cheaper, easier and safer to simply perform these massages before any form of skin penetration.

ACUPRESSURE

If you have the skills this is the simplest way to start to relax the client and develop a feel for the clients skin prior to the FCA treatment. The massage should be short, gentle and focused on relaxation and skin diagnosis rather than deep tissue techniques.

JADE ROLLERS

These crystal rollers have been produced in China for hundreds if not thousands of years. They are gentle and soothing to the client and very easy to learn. In China they were always made from nephrite jade. They can now also be bought in different crystals such as rose quartz or amethyst all of which are non porous.

They improve lymphatic drainage and microcirculation so enhancing basic skin nutrition. Given that FCA relies largely on the bodies own natural healing mechanisms to achieve results, improved skin nutrition prior to treatment can assist this process.

Used before treatments a good Jade Roller will last years with proper disinfection. It provides an affordable and effective addition to the FCA treatments. Look for a jade roller with solid brass brackets not wire as the wire is often flimsy. I have had a report from a client who was using a cheap ebay roller at home. The head fell out out and the wire, which is sharp underneath, pierced their skin through their lower eyelid. This is not something you want on your conscience or your insurance.

JADE GUA SHA

Gua Sha is an ancient Chinese Beauty tool which loosely translates as 'scraping board'. These are slightly more difficult to learn to use than the rollers but they allow you to target specific points on the face and so have a deeper therapeutic effect.

As the stimulation is deeper they should be used after the jade roller if using them together, but still before the FCA.

Some limited research has been done on Gua Sha therapy and it shows an increase in microcirculation of up to 400% following a single treatment [14]. This can certainly aid skin nutrition before a FCA treatment.

Many acupuncturists will be familiars with the plastic Gua Sha used mainly on the Back Shu and Jia Ji points. When dealing with the face I would strongly recommend crystal in preference to plastic. The slightest scratch in a plastic Gua Sha can lead to a scratch in the clients skin which they will not thank you for.

COSMETIC CUPPING

This is essentially moving cupping which most acupuncturists will be familiar with. It is performed in an upwards and outwards direction across the face.

Squeezable silicon cups are by far the best option. They can be very quickly attached and removed. This allows you to perform repeated strokes across the skin in quick succession. Unlike glass they dont get chipped. This way you never risk cutting the clients skin. Finally they don't require flames which can intimidate even the bravest of clients when applied so close to the face.

Cupping also produces all the usual benefits of massage such as increased lymphatic drainage, improved microcirculation. Additionally research has indicated that cupping may actually break up old connective tissue [15]. As discussed in the section on how FCA works, tightening of connective tissue is one of the main causes of changes in facial shape as we age.

MICRO-NEEDLE ROLLERS

These rollers were discussed briefly in the section on how FCA works. They are often also referred to as dermarollers.

Essentially they are rolled across the skin inserting very shallow micro-needles which penetrate the skin by between 0.25 - 1.0mm. By doing this they create a completely new matrix of the body's own natural collagen and elastin. It is beyond the scope of this book to explain too much about micro-needling and I have written about it extensively in previous books so I will only discuss it within the context of FCA.

These are not tools I use during an FCA treatment session, rather in particular cases I alternate FCA treatments with micro-needling. The most common reasons for this are, widespread icepick or burn scars or a very high concentrations or fine wrinkles where it is hard to target all the wrinkles individually. In most cases micro-needle rollers are also a better choice than acupuncture to assist stretch marks, cellulite and hair loss.

When using the two processes together I use micro-needling one week and FCA the next.

SUMMARY OF THE ORDER OF TREATMENT

1. Acupressure
2. Jade Roller
3. Jade Gua Sha
4. Cosmetic Cupping
5. FCA
6. Micro-needling on alternate weeks to FCA

Appendixes

APPENDIX A: PRODUCTS USED DURING TREATMENTS

For full disclosure I need to point out that some of these products are produced by White Lotus, the company I co-founded. I have spent almost 20 years studying and practicing these techniques and so have developed a range of products specifically because I believe they work best with the treatments.

Acupuncture Needles - Sieren acupuncture needles 15mm long and gauges 12 and 16.

More cosmetic acupuncture needles are entering the market constantly and the quality is improving so there are now other good choices available as well.

Swabs - Multiple Brands

Depending on where you are practicing swabs are no longer compulsory for use with acupuncture. Where possible avoid the application of alcohol to the face as it dehydrates the skin making wrinkles look worse. Also bear in mind that Muslim clients will reject any cleaning products containing ethanol.

Aftercare Serum - White Lotus Organic Green Tea facial Oil with Rejuvenating Adaptogenic Herbs

Following a treatment I ask clients to apply organic green tea oil to their faces to protect their skin and to enhance their results between treatments. I prefer oil to water based aftercare serums as they are more deeply nourishing.

Green tea oil has several major advantages over other common anti ageing oils such as jojoba or argon oil. Traditional texts record the opinion that Green tea oil 'does not block the pores'. As usual the ancient Chinese knew what they were talking about. It has been shown that green tea oil is non comedogenic so will not cause outbreaks of acne. This is very rare in an oil and research suggests this is due to its high content of linoleic acid.

The herbs added are Ren Shen (Ginseng), Huang Qi (Astragalus) and Gou Qi Zi (GoJi berries) all of which are well known adaptogenic herbs with powerful cosmetic actions on the skin.

Micro-needle Roller - White Lotus Hypoallergenic Skin Needling roller

We have used micro-needle rollers for over a decade in clinic. For the last 4 years I have only used a metal free hypoallergenic roller. The needles are made from a Biocompatible polymer and are created in one strip.

This has two advantages. Firstly they present no risk to clients who suffer from nickel allergy, an increasingly common issue. Secondly by creating the needles in one strip individual needles can never become dislodged and fall out creating risks for your clients.

Products from Chapter 8: Complementary Treatments

I use the White Lotus range of crystal rollers and Gua Sha. They are available in Jade, Rose Quartz, Tourmaline, Clear Quartz and Amethyst. Each has slightly different properties. All are delivered in a traditional silk lined box for storage and protection

For in clinic use it is better to use the large rose quartz and jade rollers that come with one larger head which is more relaxing for the client. These rollers are designed specifically for practitioners.

All White Lotus Crystal beauty tools come with a unique lifetime guarantee. This makes the addition of a crystal roller to your clinic very inexpensive. It also reflects White Lotus's belief that crystals are a precious resource that should not be treated as a single use disposable item.

White Lotus also stocks a range of Silicon cups in sizes that are ideal for the face.

APPENDIX B: TRADITIONAL EXTERNAL APPLICATION OF CHINESE HERBS

It is beyond the scope of this book to truly delve into the treasure trove that is the Chinese Pharmacopeia. I am also aware that fewer students now receive training in Chinese Herbal medicine. For these reasons I have only included some of the more important formulas for those who are interested. For anyone with a real passion for the field of Chineses external herbal medicine I highly recommend the book 'Complete External Therapies of Chinese Drugs' [16]. It is an absolute bible of external medicine preparation.

Below are some basic formulas that can be applied either as a face wash or used in a steamer which is a machine designed specifically to boil the herbs and project the steam gently onto the clients face. This helps to tonify the skin and open the pores. Up until 8 years ago we used a steamer constantly and had flasks of all our preferred herbal formulas in the clinic for daily use.

Now with the advent of better ready made preparations and due to time constraints we no longer prepare herbs fresh daily but the formulas are very effective for those with the time and patience.

Be aware that many Chinese herbs will stain clothes and you will need to be very careful in the application.

Simple Anti Aging formula for wrinkles and general signs of ageing

Ling Zhi, Ren Shen, Dang Gui, Tao Ren, Dan Shen and Si Gua in equal doses

Scars

Use the herbs Dang Gui, Bai Zhi, Tao Ren, Xing Ren, Dan Shen, Si Gua mixed with vinegar and soaked for at least 2 weeks. This needs to be applied twice a day so the clients must take it home with them

Acne

The following formula makes an excellent skin wash for all types of acne. Keep in mind that in mandarin Huang means yellow and that is exactly the colour this formula will stain your clothes if you are not careful

Use Huang Lian, Huang Bai, Huang Qin, Jin Yin Hua, Dang Gui, Chuan Xiong, Dan Shen, Tao Ren, Hong Hua and Bai Zhi in equal proportions as an external wash daily

Vitiligo

Use the ancient formula Bu Gu Zhi Ding which is 30% Bu Gu Zhi in alcohol and add a couple of blood circulating herbs such as Dang Gui and Tao Ren.

APPENDIX C: TAKING BEFORE AND AFTER PHOTOS

Before and After photos are so important for advertising now that it is vital to know how to take them correctly. You can of course rely on your clients to take them but the main problem is that clients often do not understand the importance of consistency. Photos taken in different light or with varying degrees of make up can look fake so it is usually better to do your own.

Here are several tips to improve these photos

1. Always take the photos in the same place under the same lighting conditions. Unfortunately natural light is sometimes best avoided as it varies too much.
2. A blank white wall is the ideal background.
3. A small piece of tape on the ground will help the client stand in the same place each time.
4. After photos need to be taken some time after the final treatment so the clients face is not red from the massage or acupuncture.
5. Ask the client not to wear any make up or remove it on their arrival.
6. Where possible ask the client to wear similar clothes as colour effects the appearance a lot.
7. Make sure their hair retains a similar style.

8. It is usually best to use the macro or some form of close up setting to record greater detail. Whatever setting you choose try to use the same settings for all photos.

9. Take lots of photos each time. Despite your best efforts the angles in most photos will be slightly different so having several will allow you to match up the before and after which are taken from the same angle.

10. If you can afford a tripod this will help with consistency and quality of photos.

11. Remember to take both the front side and 3/4 view when photographing the face.

Be aware you will need your clients explicit written consent to use their images in any form of advertising. Some will willingly give you permission if they are very happy with the results. Others may be happy to do so in return for a series of free treatments. As a general rule we have found that the wealthier and/or more well known your clients are, the less likely they are to want to appear in any form of cosmetic procedure advertising.

APPENDIX D - OTHER PUBLICATIONS BY THE AUTHOR

Books
2012: Holistic Microneedling
2019: Jade Roller, Gua Sha and Cosmetic Cupping

Online Courses
Holistic Microneedling
Jade Roller, Gua Sha and Cosmetic Cupping Course
Traditional Chinese Face Reading with Kamila Kingston

Academic Articles
2017: Acupuncture Today, (USA), 'Scar Reduction with Acupuncture and Microneedling'
2016: Journal of the Australian Traditional Medicine Society, (Australia) 'Microneedling and Acupuncture Facial Rejuvenation Compared'
2016: ACU (Finnland), 'Mikroneulauksen opiskelu voi autta kosmeettisen akupunktion tuloksia'

2016: Yin Yang (Switzerland), 'Ergebnisse und Profit durch Microneedling in Ihrer Klinik'

2016: Huang Ti (Netherlands), 'Cosmetische acupunctuur'

2016: The Journal of Chinese Medicine, 'Facial Cosmetic Acupuncture: An Alternative Theory for the Mechanisms Behind its Effectiveness'

2016: Journal of TCM (Spain) 'El Puso de la Vida, Acupunctura Facial Cosmetica: Un Analisis del Mecanismo Cientifico'

2012: Yin Yang SBO TCM Journal (Switzerland), 'Klassiche Chinesische Schonheitsgeheimnisse'

2012: Huang Ti Magazine (Netherlands), 'Van De Nederlandse vereniging voor acupunctuur'

2011: Journal Of Chinese Medicine, 'True Cosmetic Acupuncture still has it's roots in Traditional Chinese Medicine'

2011: The Acupuncturist, (UK), 'Medical Face Reading'

General Interest Articles

2017: Professional Beauty Australia, 'The Fundamentals of Chinese Face Reading'

2017: Well Being Magazine, 'Perfume Beauty Oils'

2016: Professional Beauty, 'Holistic Microneedling'

2016: Well Being Magazine, 'Holistic Microneedling'

2015: Guild News UK, 'Taking the Holistic Approach'

2015: Vitality Magazine, 'Skin Needling a Natural Alternative'

2013: Australian Hair and Beauty, 'Holistic Microneedling'

2012: Professional Beauty, 'Skin Needling Techniques Matter'

2012: Professional Beauty Australia, 'Holistic micro needling arrives in Australia'

2011: Vitality Magazine, British Association of Beauty therapy & Cosmetology, 'Cosmetic Acupuncture to Modern Skin Needling'

2011: Spa Australasia, 'Ancient Chinese Beauty Secrets'

2009: Wellbeing Magazine, 'Lose it with TCM'

2009: Wellbeing Magazine, '4 Chinese Beauty Secrets'

2007: Wellbeing magazine, 'Natural facelifts better than Botox'

References

1. Zhang, Q, & and Zhu, L, (1996). *Meridional Cosmetology: Report of 300 Cases with Discussion of Underlying Mechanism*. The International Journal of Clinical Acupuncture Vol 7, No 4, 401-405.

2. Choi, B., et al. (2015). Thread embedding acupuncture inhibits ultraviolet B irradiation-induced skin photoaging in hairless mice. *Evidence-Based Complementary and Alternative Medicine,* v. 2015, article ID 539172, 9p.

3. Kingston, A. (2012). Holistic Microneedling - The Manual of Natural Skin Needling.

4. Anastassakis, K. (2005). The Dermaroller™ Series. Private Paper.

5. Schwartz et al, (2006). internet paper. Abstract reflections about COLLAGEN-INDUCTION-THERAPY (CIT) A Hypothesis for the Mechanism of Action of Collagen Induction Therapy (CIT) using Micro-Needles. 1st edition February 2006.

6. Fernandes, D. (2005). Minimally Invasive Percutaneous Collagen Induction. *Oral Maxilla Facial Surg Clinical.*

7. Kim, T. Y. (2013). Trend Analysis of Facial Cosmetic Acupuncture Study based on the Korean Traditional Medicine. *The Acupuncture.* 30(5):125-137.

8. LI, P., Qiu, T. &Qin, C. (2015). Efficiency of Acupuncture for Bells Palsy: A Systemic Review and Meta Analysis of Random Controlled Trials. *PLoS One.* May 14: 10(5).

9. C. L. Louarn, D. Buthiau, and J. Buis. (2007). Structural aging: the facial recurve concept. *Aesthetic Plastic Surgery.* vol. 31, no. 3, pp. 213–218.

10. Younghee, Y. Sehyun, K. Minhee, K. KyuSeok, K. Jeong-Su, P. and Inhwa, C. (2013). Effect of Facial Cosmetic Acupuncture on Facial Elasticity: An Open-Label, Single-Arm Pilot Study. *Evidence-Based Complementary and Alternative Medicine.* Volume 2013.

11. Hwang DS, Song JH, Kim YS, Lee KS. (2008). The Changes of Facial Temperature by Miso Facial Rejuvenation Acupuncture: A Case Study. *The Journal of Korean Acupuncture & Moxibustion Society.* 25;1. 89–95.

12. Kim, M. S. (2013). A Study on Cosmetic Acupuncture Through Anatomy and Physiology Interpretation. *Korean Journal of Acupuncture.* Volume 30, Issue 3, pp.171-177.

13. Orentreich, D.S. Orentreich, N. (1995). Subcutaneous incisionless (subcision) surgery for the correction of depressed scars and wrinkles. *Dermatol Surg.* Jun21(6). 543-549.

14. Nielsen A, et al. (2007). The effect of Gua Sha treatment on the microcirculation of surface tissue: a pilot study in healthy subjects. *Explore* (NY). Sep-Oct;3(5):456-66.

15. Cao, H., Han, M., Li, X., et al. Clinical research evidence of cupping therapy in China: a systematic literature review. *BMC Complementary and Alternative Medicine*. 2010;10:70.

16. Xu, X. (1998). Complete External Therapies of Chinese Drugs Hardcover. *Foreign Languages Press.*

Thank you for taking the time to read this book. I genuinely hope it was useful to you.

If you would like to learn more please visit our websites and apply the code thanksagain to receive a 20% discount off the range of books and online courses.

For those who would like to access the full video content of the White Lotus Advanced Cosmetic Acupuncture Online Course please enter the code FCA50 to receive a 50% discount on this course.

Finally White Lotus offers a full range of cosmetic in clinic products to assist busy acupuncturists. Please contact us directly to apply for a wholesale account.

International Customers

www.whitelotusbeauty.com
info@whitelotusbeauty.com

Australian Customers

www.whitelotus.com.au
info@whitelotus.com.au

CPSIA information can be obtained
at www.ICGtesting.com
Printed in the USA
LVHW071340121121
703167LV00001B/4

* 9 7 8 0 6 4 6 8 2 8 0 2 2 *